Praise for *Idiopathic Scoliosis*

"This infinitely readable and well-researched book does an amazing job of explaining everything about idiopathic scoliosis. It provides meaningful insights into scoliosis not only for patients and their families and friends but also for health care providers at all levels who have an interest in, or care for, these patients. I was particularly impressed with the patient stories interwoven with scientific information, bringing a much-appreciated, warm, human element to the book. Bravo to the team at Gillette."

BENJAMIN D. ROYE, Pediatric Orthopedic Surgeon, Morgan Stanley Children's Hospital of New York; Richard T. Arkwright–St. Giles Foundation Associate Professor, Orthopedic Surgery, Columbia University, US

"This book is great for anyone on this journey! Our daughter was diagnosed with juvenile idiopathic scoliosis right before she started kindergarten, and we were so worried and overwhelmed, and had so many questions. We wish we had this book during that time as it answers so many questions. We still have many questions and this book helps us pave a path today and for the future."

AMBER MARLATT, Parent of daughter with juvenile idiopathic scoliosis, US

"Written by experts at Gillette Children's, Idiopathic Scoliosis *is both a source of information and psychological support for families and patients with scoliosis. The information in the book is comprehensive and clear, but most important and enjoyable are the clinical stories of patients and families who have benefited from the expertise of the spine experts at Gillette Children's. Readers are provided with an objective picture of the pathology and its treatment without false illusions or easy enthusiasm. The clear drawings help readers understand even the most technical and complex aspects of idiopathic scoliosis, supported by up-to-date references. The book is a must-read!"*

FEDERICO CANAVESE, Head, Orthopedic and Traumatology Department, IRCCS Giannina Gaslini Institute, Genoa; Professor of Pediatric Orthopedics, University of Genoa, Italy

"This easy-to-read book will be an invaluable resource for parents who are new to dealing with a child or adolescent who has been diagnosed with scoliosis and who need comprehensive and validated information about the condition and treatment options. I wish this book had been available when I was faced with my teenage daughter being diagnosed with scoliosis."

EILISH MCLOUGHLIN, Parent of daughter with adolescent idiopathic scoliosis, UK

T0325377

"*This book,* Idiopathic Scoliosis, *is a comprehensive, well-structured, easily readable resource. The information is presented in a very straightforward, logical, and understandable manner, and it is well referenced and accompanied by helpful photographs and diagrams. The input from actual patients and families provides a very personal perspective of the scoliosis journey.*"

BRIAN SMITH, L.E. Simmons Chief of Orthopaedics, Texas Children's Hospital; Professor of Orthopaedics, Baylor College of Medicine, US

"*The expert staff from Gillette Children's have done a remarkable job in creating a comprehensive review for families of children with idiopathic scoliosis. Family journeys are interwoven with an up-to-date review of the causes of scoliosis and modern treatment options. Discussion of nonsurgical and surgical treatments are balanced, allowing families to better prepare for discussions with their care team. Unique to this book is guidance on how best to transition to care when patients age out of pediatric health care.*"

SUMEET GARG, Pediatric Orthopaedic Surgeon, Children's Hospital Colorado; Professor of Orthopaedic Surgery, University of Colorado School of Medicine, US

"*This book is one of the best resources available for patients and families to understand scoliosis and its treatment, both nonsurgical and surgical. The real-life stories of patients and families allow newly diagnosed scoliosis patients to understand the condition and its treatment and—more importantly—to let them know they are not alone. It covers the entire treatment landscape, with the latest techniques supported by the most recent published scientific data. I highly recommend this book to anyone who is affected by scoliosis and wants to educate themselves with the most complete resource in an easy-to-read format.*"

ROBERT H. CHO, Chief of Staff, Shriners Children's Southern California, Pediatric Orthopedic Surgeon, Pediatric Spine Surgeon, UCLA Clinical Assistant Professor, US

"*The visuals and organization are very helpful in understanding signs, symptoms, and possible treatment plans of scoliosis. As a patient, I found the inclusion of personal narratives throughout the book comforted me about the diagnosis and the care I would be provided with.*"

ISABELLA VERMEDAHL, Adult with adolescent idiopathic scoliosis, US

"*This comprehensive book on idiopathic scoliosis for parents of children with the condition is a gem for its clarity in explaining complex medical concepts in accessible language. It clearly lays out the chronological progression of scoliosis treatment, guiding parents through each step with precision and care. The accuracy of the information presented instills confidence in readers, making it a trusted resource for understanding and managing scoliosis effectively. This book is a must-have for parents seeking reliable information and support on navigating the challenges of scoliosis.*"

DAVID P. MOORE, Consultant Orthopaedic Surgeon, Children's Health Ireland

"The spine team at Gillette has done a nice job of putting together a comprehensive but accessible book on idiopathic scoliosis. The patient story is an excellent companion to the clinical information in the book. The pictures and diagrams are helpful and easy to understand. A great read!"

KEITH D. BALDWIN, Director of Orthopedic Trauma, Associate Professor, Children's Hospital of Philadelphia, US

"This unique resource provides not only information about the treatment of scoliosis but also the perspective of the patient and parent. Getting a diagnosis of scoliosis can often seem daunting. Yet as providers treating this condition, we see that even in severe cases where a spinal fusion is ultimately needed, patients typically return to full sports and activities. This book will be a welcome companion to many as they embark on their scoliosis journey."

LINDSAY M. ANDRAS, Director of Spine and Vice Chief of Orthopedics, Children's Hospital Los Angeles, US

"This book is as up-to-date and inclusive as a textbook written for medical professionals while being as easily readable as a novel for children with scoliosis and their families. Reading the story of Lila on her journey will alleviate the fears of children with scoliosis, and following her mother's testimonials step by step will soothe families' anxieties. This brief but comprehensive guide is a light to illuminate the way for both children diagnosed with scoliosis and their families, and it is an indispensable source of comfort for all scoliosis patients. Congratulations to the authors."

MUHARREM YAZICI, Professor of Orthopaedics Children's Orthopaedics and Spine Center, Ankara, Turkey; Past President European Pediatric Orthopedic Society; Past President Scoliosis Research Society

IDIOPATHIC SCOLIOSIS

IDIOPATHIC SCOLIOSIS

Understanding and
managing the condition:
A practical guide
for families

Tenner J. Guillaume, MD
Walter H. Truong, MD
Danielle Harding, PA-C
Michaela Hingtgen, MS
The VanGoethem Family

Edited by
Lily Collison, MA, MSc
Elizabeth R. Boyer, PhD
Tom F. Novacheck, MD
GILLETTE CHILDREN'S

Copyright © 2024 Gillette Children's Healthcare Press

All rights reserved. No part of this publication may be reproduced, stored in a retrieval system, or transmitted in any form or by any means, without the prior written consent of Gillette Children's Healthcare Press.

Gillette Children's Healthcare Press
200 University Avenue East
St Paul, MN 55101
www.GilletteChildrensHealthcarePress.org
HealthcarePress@gillettechildrens.com

ISBN 978-1-952181-11-5 (paperback)
ISBN 978-1-952181-12-2 (e-book)
LIBRARY OF CONGRESS CONTROL NUMBER 2024941534

COPYEDITING BY Ruth Wilson
ORIGINAL ILLUSTRATIONS BY Olwyn Roche
COVER AND INTERIOR DESIGN BY Jazmin Welch
PROOFREADING BY Ruth Wilson
INDEX BY Audrey McClellan

Printed by Hobbs the Printers Ltd, Totton, Hampshire, UK

For information about distribution or special discounts for bulk purchases, please contact:
Mac Keith Press
2nd Floor, Rankin Building
139-143 Bermondsey Street
London, SE1 3UW
www.mackeith.co.uk
admin@mackeith.co.uk

The views and opinions expressed herein are those of the authors and Gillette Children's Healthcare Press and do not necessarily represent those of Mac Keith Press.

To individuals and families whose lives are affected by these conditions, to professionals who serve our community, and to all clinicians and researchers who push the knowledge base forward, we hope the books in this Healthcare Series serve you very well.

All proceeds from the books in this series at Gillette Children's go to research.

*All information contained in this book is for educational purposes only. For specific medical advice and treatment, please consult a qualified health care professional.
The information in this book is not intended as a substitute for consultation with your health care professional.*

Contents

Authors and Editors

Tenner J. Guillaume, MD, Spine Surgeon and Chair of Spine Institute, Gillette Children's

Walter H. Truong, MD, Pediatric Orthopedic Surgeon, Gillette Children's; Associate Professor of Orthopedics, University of Minnesota

Danielle Harding, PA-C, MPAS-Pediatrics, Physician Assistant, Gillette Children's

Michaela Hingtgen, MS, Principal Writer, Gillette Children's Healthcare Press

The VanGoethem Family

Lily Collison, MA, MSc, Program Director, Gillette Children's Healthcare Press

Elizabeth R. Boyer, PhD, Clinical Scientist, Gillette Children's

Tom F. Novacheck, MD, Medical Director of Integrated Care Services, Gillette Children's; Professor of Orthopedics, University of Minnesota; and Past President, American Academy for Cerebral Palsy and Developmental Medicine

Series Foreword

You hold in your hands one book in the Gillette Children's Healthcare Series. This series was inspired by multiple factors.

It started with Lily Collison writing the first book in the series, *Spastic Diplegia–Bilateral Cerebral Palsy*. Lily has a background in medical science and is the parent of a now adult son who has spastic diplegia. Lily was convincing at the time about the value of such a book, and with the publication of that book in 2020, Gillette Children's became one of the first children's hospitals in the world to set up its own publishing arm—Gillette Children's Healthcare Press. *Spastic Diplegia–Bilateral Cerebral Palsy* received very positive reviews from both families and professionals and achieved strong sales. Unsolicited requests came in from diverse organizations across the globe for translation rights, and feedback from families told us there was a demand for books relevant to other conditions.

We listened.

We were convinced of the value of expanding from one book into a series to reflect Gillette Children's strong commitment to worldwide education. In 2021, Lily joined the press as Program Director, and very quickly, Gillette Children's formed teams to write the Healthcare Series. The series includes, in order of publication:

- *Craniosynostosis*
- *Idiopathic Scoliosis*
- *Spastic Hemiplegia—Unilateral Cerebral Palsy*
- *Spastic Quadriplegia—Bilateral Cerebral Palsy*
- *Spastic Diplegia—Bilateral Cerebral Palsy, second edition*
- *Epilepsy*
- *Spina Bifida*
- *Osteogenesis Imperfecta*
- *Scoliosis—Congenital, Neuromuscular, Syndromic, and Other Causes*

The books address each condition detailing both the medical and human story.

Mac Keith Press, long-time publisher of books on disability and the journal *Developmental Medicine and Child Neurology,* is co-publishing this series with Gillette Children's Healthcare Press.

Families and professionals working well together is key to best management of any condition. The parent is the expert of their child while the professional is the expert of the condition. These books underscore the importance of that family and professional partnership. For each title in the series, medical professionals at Gillette Children's have led the writing, and families contributed the lived experience.

These books have been written in the United States with an international lens and citing international research. However, there isn't always strong evidence to create consensus in medicine, so others may take a different view.

We hope you find the book you hold in your hands to be of great value. We collectively strive to optimize outcomes for children, adolescents, and adults living with these childhood-acquired and largely lifelong conditions.

Dr. Tom F. Novacheck

Series Introduction

The Healthcare Series seeks to optimize outcomes for those who live with childhood-acquired physical and/or neurological conditions. The conditions addressed in this series of books are complex and often have many associated challenges. Although the books focus on the biomedical aspects of each condition, we endeavor to address each condition as holistically as possible. Since the majority of people with these conditions have them for life, the life course is addressed including transition and aging issues.

Who are these books for?

These books are written for an international audience. They are primarily written for parents of young children, but also for adolescents and adults who have the condition. They are written for members of multidisciplinary teams and researchers. Finally, they are written for others, including extended family members, teachers, and students taking courses in the fields of medicine, allied health care, and education.

A worldview

The books in the series focus on evidence-based best practice, which we acknowledge is not available everywhere. It is mostly available in high-income countries (at least in urban areas, though even there, not always), but many families live away from centers of good care.

We also acknowledge that the majority of people with disabilities live in low- and middle-income countries. Improving the lives of all those with disabilities across the globe is an important goal. Developing scalable, affordable interventions is a crucial step toward achieving this. Nonetheless, the best interventions will fail if we do not first address the social determinants of health—the economic, social, and environmental conditions in which people live that shape their overall health and well-being.

No family reading these books should ever feel they have failed their child. We all struggle to do our best for our children within the limitations of our various resources and situations. Indeed, the advocacy role these books may play may help families and professionals lobby in unison for best care.

International Classification of Functioning, Disability and Health

The writing of the series of books has been informed by the International Classification of Functioning, Disability and Health (ICF).[1] The framework explains the impact of a health condition at different levels and how those levels are interconnected. It tells us to look at the full picture—to look at the person with a disability in their life situation.

The framework shows that every human being can experience a decrease in health and thereby experience some disability. It is not something that happens only to a minority of people. The ICF thus "mainstreams" disability and recognizes it as a widespread human experience.

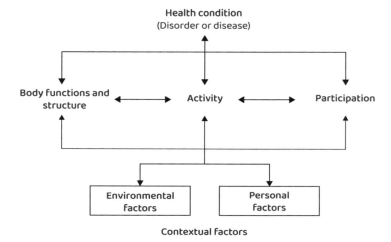

International Classification of Functioning, Disability and Health (ICF). Reproduced with kind permission from WHO.

In health care, there has been a shift away from focusing almost exclusively on correcting issues that cause the individual's functional problems to focusing also on the individual's activity and participation. These books embrace maximizing participation for all people living with disability.

The Family

For simplicity, throughout the series we refer to "parents" and "children"; we acknowledge, however, that family structures vary. "Parent" is used as a generic term that includes grandparents, relatives, and carers (caregivers) who are raising a child. Throughout the series, we refer to male and female as the biologic sex assigned at birth. We acknowledge that this does not equate to gender identity or sexual orientation, and we respect the individuality of each person. Throughout the series we have included both "person with disability" and "disabled person," recognizing that both terms are used.

Caring for a child with a disability can be challenging and overwhelming. Having a strong social support system in place can make a difference. For the parent, balancing the needs of the child with a disability with the needs of siblings—while also meeting employment demands, nurturing a relationship with a significant other, and caring for aging parents—can sometimes feel like an enormous juggling act. Siblings may feel neglected or overlooked because of the increased attention given to the disabled child. It is crucial for parents to allocate time and resources to ensure that siblings feel valued and included in the family dynamics. Engaging siblings in the care and support of the disabled child can help foster a sense of unity and empathy within the family.

A particular challenge for a child and adolescent who has a disability, and their parent, is balancing school attendance (for both academic and social purposes) with clinical appointments and surgery. Appointments outside of school hours are encouraged. School is important because the cognitive and social abilities developed there help maximize employment opportunities when employment is a realistic goal. Indeed, technology has eliminated barriers and created opportunities that did not exist even 10 years ago.

Parents also need to find a way to prioritize self-care. Neglecting their own well-being can have detrimental effects on their mental and physical health. Think of the safety advice on an airplane: you are told that you must put on your own oxygen mask before putting on your child's. It's the same when caring for a child with a disability; parents need to take care of themselves in order to effectively care for their child *and* family. Friends, support groups, or mental health professionals can provide an outlet for parents to express their emotions, gain valuable insights, and find solace in knowing that they are not alone in their journey.

For those of you reading this book who have the condition, we hope this book gives you insights into its many nuances and complexities, acknowledges you as an expert in your own care, and provides a road-map and framework for you to advocate for your needs.

Last words

This series of books seeks to be an invaluable educational resource. All proceeds from the series at Gillette Children's go to research.

Chapter 1

Scoliosis

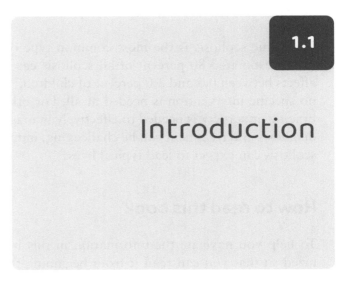

Introduction

The secret of getting ahead is getting started.
Mark Twain

If you were to look up the definition of scoliosis (pronounced SKOL-ee-oh-sis, with the capital letters showing the emphasis on that syllable), you would find many sources defining it as a sideways curvature of the spine. This is generally correct, but a more accurate definition of scoliosis is a condition in which there is an atypical three-dimensional curvature and rotation of the spine.[2]

There are many types of scoliosis with varied causes. This book focuses on a type of scoliosis called idiopathic scoliosis. The term "idiopathic" is defined as "relating to a disease of unknown cause," and it is used in the context of many medical conditions for which the cause is unclear or unknown. Idiopathic scoliosis is, therefore, scoliosis that develops from an unknown cause. There are a few theories about the mechanisms that cause the spine to grow in a curved and rotated fashion in idiopathic scoliosis; perhaps the most accepted is that the front of the spine grows faster than the back of the spine.[3] As the front grows faster, the spine begins to rotate, twist, and curve to the side. However, ultimately, it is unclear what causes these mechanisms to develop in the first place. Individuals with idiopathic scoliosis are otherwise typically developing with no related underlying medical conditions.

Idiopathic scoliosis is the most common type of scoliosis, accounting for an estimated 80 percent of all scoliosis cases.[4] Idiopathic scoliosis affects between 0.5 and 3.0 percent of children.[3] For the large majority, no specific intervention is needed at all. For others, treatment such as bracing or surgery is needed to effectively manage the condition. While diagnosis and treatment can be challenging, individuals with idiopathic scoliosis can expect to lead typical lives.

How to read this book

To help you navigate the information in this book, it has been organized so that you can read it from beginning to end or, alternatively, dip into different sections and chapters independently. Because much of the information builds on previous sections and chapters, it is best to first read the book in its entirety to get an overall sense of the condition. After that, you can return to the parts that are relevant to you, knowing that you can ignore other sections or revisit them if and when they become relevant.

This chapter addresses the overall condition of scoliosis. Chapter 2 addresses idiopathic scoliosis, and Chapters 3 and 4 address treatment of idiopathic scoliosis. Chapter 5 looks at idiopathic scoliosis in adulthood.

Throughout the book, medical information is interspersed with personal lived experience. Orange boxes highlight the personal story of Lila VanGoethem, age 15, and her mother, Tana. Both have written about their experiences with Lila's scoliosis. Chapter 6 is devoted to vignettes from other individuals and families around the globe. Chapter 7 provides further reading and research.

At the back of the book, you'll find a glossary of key terms. A companion website for this book is available at www.GilletteChildrensHealthcare Press.org. A QR code to access **Useful web resources** is included below.

Tana

Lila was 12 years old when she was diagnosed, although her pediatrician had been monitoring her for potential scoliosis for years. Shortly after her diagnosis, Lila was fitted for a brace, and eventually she had both a daytime and a nighttime brace. While Lila wore her braces regularly for about 18 months, her curve continued to worsen. With the guidance of her doctor, we made the decision for Lila to have vertebral body tethering surgery. Today, nearly 20 months after her surgery, Lila is a happy, healthy, very active teenager. We are thankful for the care from her doctor and the care team, and grateful for Lila to have had the opportunity to have this surgery. While Lila is still a growing teen and her scoliosis journey continues, we are confident in our decisions and believe we have done everything we can to support her.

I encourage all parents and caregivers to ask questions of your care team and take in all the information (buying this book is a great step in that direction). Once you have all the information and know your options, use that knowledge to make the best decision available for your child at the time. No one knows your child as well as you do. If your child is able to weigh in on that decision, allow them to also hear the information and ask questions. Stay positive, and be brave with them through all phases of the journey. Wearing a brace in middle school is a very brave thing for a teen to do. As parents and caregivers, we can support our child by reassuring them that this time in their life does not define them, and that having to wear a brace is most often a phase. Ask your child what they need to get through this time. It may be as simple as wearing a large sweatshirt over their brace at school. And have hope. Lila's scoliosis diagnosis has been (ironically) such a positive part of her life story. It has given her fortitude, confidence, and a positive attitude.

Lila

I would tell a kid who recently got diagnosed with scoliosis to stay strong and to not focus on it too much. I thought when I got diagnosed that it was scary, and I didn't know what was going to happen to me. But it ended up not being scary at all because of all the amazing doctors (and my family) to help me through it. I always felt better knowing that although this was really hard to deal with right now, and it's an experience that most kids don't have to go through, it will be over quicker than you realize and you will feel better about your back in the end. Every kid that I ended up eventually telling about my back braces afterwards said that they were sorry I had to go through that and they are amazed at how well I did while I was diagnosed, and now.

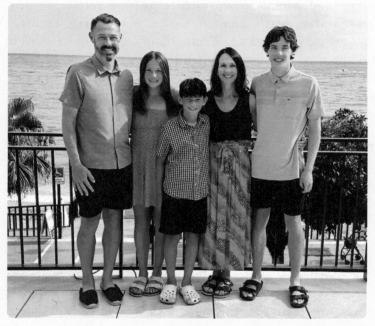

The VanGoethem family. Lila (left middle) and her mother, Tana (right middle).

USEFUL WEB RESOURCES

Understanding the spine

Knowing yourself is the beginning of all wisdom.
Aristotle

The spine has many names. You may hear people refer to it as the backbone, vertebral column, or spinal column. All these names refer to the same skeletal, or bony, structure that surrounds the spinal cord. In this book, "spine" is used consistently to describe this skeletal structure.

To understand scoliosis, it's important to first have a basic understanding of the spine itself: its function and anatomy, typical curvature, and development.

Spine function and anatomy

The spine serves four important functions:

- Protecting the spinal cord
- Serving as an attachment point for the ribs and supporting muscles and ligaments
- Supporting the weight of the body
- Providing points of movement for the head and torso

The spine consists of vertebrae and intervertebral discs. Key parts are described below and are illustrated in Figure 1.2.1.

- **Vertebrae** are bony structures with a hole in the middle for the spinal cord to pass through (this hole is also referred to as the spinal canal).
  - The **vertebral body** is the column-shaped part of the vertebra that bears the majority of the load or body weight.
  - The **pedicles** are bony bridges located on the left and right sides of each vertebra, connecting the front of the vertebra to the back of the vertebra.
  - The **facet joints** are the areas along the back of the spine where two vertebrae meet. Like most joints in the body, facet joints provide movement and flexibility to the spine.
  - The **intervertebral foramen** is the opening between each vertebra that allows nerves to branch off the spinal cord and travel to other parts of the body.
- **Intervertebral discs** are cartilage structures that sit between vertebral bodies. The gelatinous material in the center offers shock absorption during movement, as well as increased flexibility.

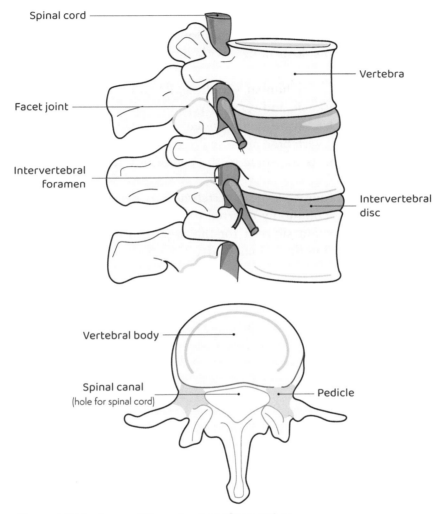

Figure 1.2.1 Anatomy of the spine and of a vertebra.

Humans typically have 33 vertebrae, which are commonly grouped into five regions of the spine: cervical, thoracic, lumbar, sacral, and coccygeal. Each region has unique characteristics and functionality. The facet joints between vertebrae are oriented differently throughout the spine, allowing for different types of motion in each region. These regions of the spine are shown in Figure 1.2.2.

- **Cervical:** There are seven cervical vertebrae, C1 to C7. These vertebrae are quite small, support the weight of the head, and enable head and neck movement.

- **Thoracic:** There are 12 thoracic vertebrae, T1 to T12. These vertebrae support the attached ribs and allow for rotation of the torso as well as side-to-side bending, with limited movement forward and backward.
- **Lumbar:** There are five lumbar vertebrae, L1 to L5. They are much larger than the thoracic and cervical vertebrae and allow for bending forward and backward, with limited side-to-side bending.
- **Sacral:** Five sacral vertebrae are fused together to form the sacrum. The sacrum connects the spine to the pelvis and provides strength and stability.
- **Coccygeal:** The four coccygeal vertebrae are partially fused and form the coccyx, commonly referred to as the tail bone. While the coccyx provides slight support for the organs in the pelvis, it has very little function in the human body.

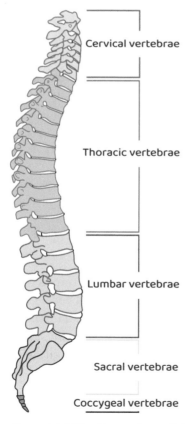

Cervical vertebrae

Thoracic vertebrae

Lumbar vertebrae

Sacral vertebrae

Coccygeal vertebrae

Figure 1.2.2 The five regions of the spine.

Typical spine curvature

In addition to the different structures of vertebrae and types of motion in each region of the spine, each region has a unique typical curvature. The typical curvature is also referred to as the natural curvature of the spine. When looking at a person straight on, the spine appears straight. In contrast, when looking at the side view of a person, the spine has distinct curvature. The direction of these curvatures is defined using two key terms: lordosis and kyphosis.

- **Lordosis** is an inward curvature, arching toward the center of the body.
- **Kyphosis** is an outward curvature, rounding away from the center of the body.

Figure 1.2.3 shows the typical curvature of the spine: a slight cervical lordosis, thoracic kyphosis, lumbar lordosis, and sacral kyphosis. These curvatures represent the body's preferred alignment when in an upright position and allow for an equal distribution of weight across the spine.[5]

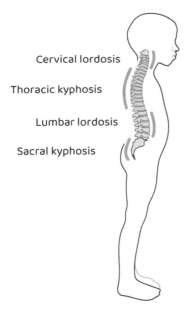

Cervical lordosis

Thoracic kyphosis

Lumbar lordosis

Sacral kyphosis

Figure 1.2.3 The typical (natural) curvature of the spine.

Spine development

Vertebrae begin to develop early in pregnancy. Around three weeks after conception, the vertebrae and ribs of the developing baby begin to form from cartilage that is later replaced by bone cells. This process of cartilage being replaced by bone cells, also called ossification, continues until about age 25.[6]

The spinal curvatures also begin developing during pregnancy and continue through childhood. Kyphosis curvatures form while the baby lies in a naturally curved (fetal) position in the uterus. In contrast, the lordotic curvatures form later in childhood: cervical lordotic curvature when babies begin to support the weight of their head, and lumbar lordotic curvature when children begin to support their body weight through standing. Because of when these curvatures develop, kyphosis is often referred to as a "primary" curvature of the spine, and lordosis as a "secondary" curvature.

Anatomical planes

Our bodies exist in three dimensions of space. Anatomical planes are imaginary divisions of the body. Anatomical planes are especially useful when discussing the spine because the typical curvature of the spine differs in each plane. Figure 1.2.4 shows the body divided into cross-sections in three anatomical planes:

- **The axial plane** separates the upper and lower halves of the body. As the observer looking at the axial plane of the body, you are above a standing person, looking down at the top of their head. This is also referred to as the transverse plane. The term "axial plane" is used throughout this book.
- **The coronal plane** separates the front and back of the body. As the observer looking at the coronal plane of the body, you are looking at a person who is facing you straight on or away from you. This is also referred to as the frontal plane. The term "coronal plane" is used throughout this book.
- **The sagittal plane** separates the left and right sides of the body. As the observer looking at the sagittal plane of the body, you are

looking at the side view of a person. This is also referred to as the lateral plane. The term "sagittal plane" is used throughout this book.

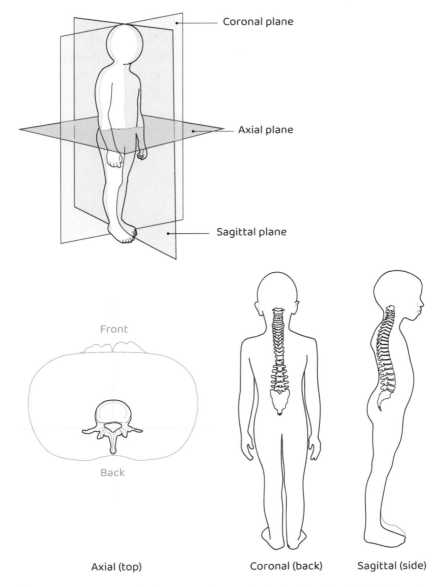

Figure 1.2.4 Anatomical planes on a human body (top) and applied to the spine (bottom).

A typical spine when viewed in the coronal plane is straight but has a notable curvature in the sagittal plane (see Figure 1.2.4). The coronal view shown in the figure is of a person facing directly away from you and shows the back of the person's body. A spine specialist will often examine the spine (in person and in X-rays) from the back. **Note:** "Spine specialist" refers to an orthopedic spine surgeon or advanced practice provider.* At some medical centers, a neurosurgeon may manage the individual's scoliosis instead of an orthopedic spine surgeon.

---

* In the US, an advanced practice provider (APP) is a health care provider who is not a physician but who performs medical activities typically performed by a physician. This includes a physician assistant (PA) and a nurse practitioner (NP), both medical professionals who complete graduate schooling, have greater medical privileges than nurses, and work on the care team. These roles may have different titles in other countries.

Atypical spine curvatures

Divide each difficulty into as many parts as is
feasible and necessary to resolve it.
René Descartes

There are many conditions that can affect the anatomy, curvatures, and development of the spine, leading to other atypical spine curvatures, not just scoliosis. Because these other atypical spine curvatures may impact care plans, they are included in this book.

Identifying the cause of atypical spine curvatures can be challenging. What they have in common is that they disrupt the typical curvatures of the spine in one, two, or all three anatomical planes. Atypical spine curvatures range from mild to severe and can occur in infants, children, adolescents, and adults. Atypical spine curvatures may be present from birth (congenital), may develop while the spine is growing, or may develop after an event such as an infection, surgery, or trauma.

These atypical curvatures are hyper- or hypokyphosis, hyper- or hypolordosis, and scoliosis. The first two (kyphosis and lordosis) represent curvatures in the sagittal plane and are *not* scoliosis.

Hyper- or hypokyphosis

Kyphosis is an outward curvature of the spine, rounding away from the center of the body. This curvature is visible only in the sagittal plane. When upright, a typical spine has slight kyphosis in the thoracic and sacral regions. When the amount of kyphosis is atypical, the term "kyphosis" is assigned either the prefix "hyper," meaning *above* typical, or "hypo," meaning *below* typical. Hyperkyphosis indicates excessive rounding of the spine, typically in the thoracic region (Figure 1.3.1). Hypokyphosis indicates a loss of kyphosis and the presentation of an abnormally straight or flat spine. Again, hyperkyphosis and hypokyphosis are *not* scoliosis.

Hyperkyphosis can have many different causes ranging from structural differences in the vertebrae to an individual standing with slouched or hunched posture. Hypokyphosis is often associated with idiopathic scoliosis. Recall the theory that idiopathic scoliosis is due to overgrowth of the front of the spine relative to the back of the spine. As the front of the spine grows, becoming longer than the back of the spine, it can result in hypokyphosis in some individuals with idiopathic scoliosis.

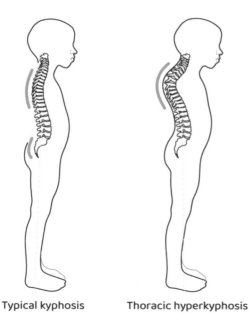

Typical kyphosis   Thoracic hyperkyphosis

Figure 1.3.1. Typical kyphosis and thoracic hyperkyphosis.

Hyper- or hypolordosis

Lordosis is an inward curvature of the spine, arching toward the center of the body. This curvature is visible only in the sagittal plane. When upright, a typical spine has lordosis in the cervical and lumbar regions. In the same manner as kyphosis, when the amount of lordosis is atypical, the prefixes "hyper" or "hypo" are used.

Hyperlordosis indicates excessive arching of the spine, typically in the lumbar region, but this can also develop in the cervical region (Figure 1.3.2). This excessive arching in the lumbar region is sometimes described as having a swayback appearance. Hypolordosis indicates a loss of lordosis and the presentation of an abnormally straight or flat spine, typically in the lumbar region. Again, hyperlordosis and hypolordosis are *not* scoliosis.

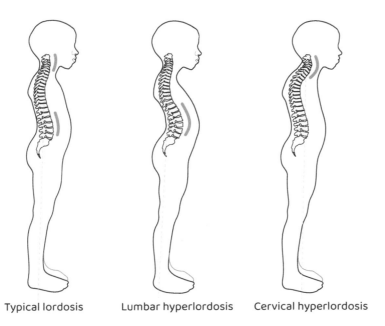

Typical lordosis   Lumbar hyperlordosis   Cervical hyperlordosis

Figure 1.3.2 Typical lordosis contrasted with hyperlordosis in the lumbar and cervical regions of the spine.

Hyperlordosis has many possible causes ranging from weak muscles surrounding the stomach and lower back to injuries to the spine to differences in how the bones were formed prior to birth (such as a wedged instead of a rectangular vertebra). Similarly, hypolordosis has other causes such as structural differences in the vertebrae.

See Appendix 1 (online) for a detailed list of causes of hyper- and hypo-kyphosis, and hyper- and hypolordosis.

Scoliosis

Scoliosis is characterized by rotation (twisting) in the axial plane, side-ways curvature in the coronal plane, and flattening or exaggeration of curvature in the sagittal plane (Figure 1.3.3). While the largest change from typical spine curvature occurs in the coronal plane, scoliosis is described as three dimensional because it affects the spine in all three anatomical planes.

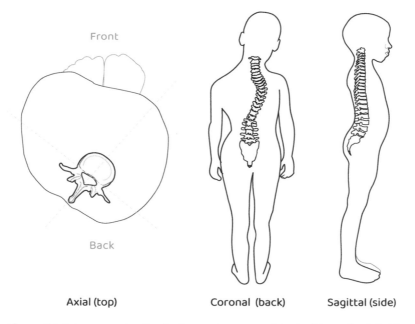

Axial (top)   Coronal (back)   Sagittal (side)

Figure 1.3.3 An example of spinal curvature associated with scoliosis in the axial, coronal, and sagittal planes.

Classification of scoliosis

Two roads diverged in a wood and I—
I took the one less traveled by,
And that has made all the difference.
Robert Frost

The two most common factors by which scoliosis is classified are cause and age at diagnosis. Classification is useful for describing someone's scoliosis and how it may progress. It also helps medical professionals make care decisions and recommend treatment options.

By cause

There are five types of scoliosis classified by cause:

- Idiopathic
- Congenital
- Neuromuscular
- Syndromic
- Other

See Table 1.4.1 for details.

Table 1.4.1 Classification of scoliosis based on cause

TYPE	CAUSE
Idiopathic	The term "idiopathic" means there is no known cause. With idiopathic scoliosis, the spine grows in a curved and rotated fashion for unknown reasons.
Congenital	The term "congenital" means present from birth. Congenital scoliosis is caused by errors in vertebral development. The child is born with an atypical spine (atypical vertebrae and/or atypical intervertebral discs) that can cause atypical growth of the spine, resulting in scoliosis.
Neuromuscular	The term "neuromuscular" means a condition involving the nervous system and/or muscles; it includes conditions such as cerebral palsy. Because nerves and/or muscles are affected, it can prevent the body from being able to physically support a growing spine, resulting in scoliosis.
Syndromic	The term "syndromic" means a group of symptoms that consistently occur together. Syndromic scoliosis is caused by a syndrome, such as Marfan syndrome or Down syndrome. These conditions can cause connective tissue (e.g., bone, blood vessels, cartilage, ligaments, tendons) to weaken, resulting in scoliosis.
Other	Other causes of scoliosis include conditions such as neural axis abnormalities, which are atypical structures within the central nervous system (brain and/or spinal cord) that can impact the growth of the spine.

By age of diagnosis

Scoliosis can also be classified by the age of diagnosis. One age-based classification is early-onset scoliosis (EOS), which is defined as scoliosis that is diagnosed prior to 10 years of age, regardless of cause or type.

There are also age-based classifications specific to idiopathic scoliosis:

- Infantile idiopathic scoliosis (IIS)—age of diagnosis 0 to 3 years
- Juvenile idiopathic scoliosis (JIS)—age of diagnosis 4 to 9 years
- Adolescent idiopathic scoliosis (AIS)—age of diagnosis 10 to 18 years

Diagnosis of scoliosis

Faith is taking the first step even when
you don't see the whole staircase.
Martin Luther King Jr.

Individuals can be diagnosed with scoliosis at any age. However, especially in the case of idiopathic scoliosis, it is most commonly diagnosed between the ages of 10 and 15.[7] Children enter their pubertal growth spurt at this age, and this rapid growth is associated with an increased risk of scoliosis curve progression (i.e., getting larger). The larger a curve becomes, the more noticeable the signs and symptoms become to an individual, parent, and/or medical professional.

- A **sign** is what can be seen by observing the individual (e.g., a visibly curved spine).
- A **symptom** is what the individual describes as experiencing due to the condition (e.g., back pain).

The typical diagnostic journey for children and adolescents with idiopathic scoliosis, from first detection through to the first appointment with a spine specialist, is described next. Of course, a "typical" journey will not apply to all families; the diagnostic journey may look very different depending on the country the family lives in or hospital or treatment center they are attending.

First detection

Typically, scoliosis is first noted by the child, parent, or the primary care provider.* The following changes in a child's appearance are signs of scoliosis:[8]

- One shoulder being higher than the other
- A curved spine that looks like an "S" or "C" rather than a straight line down the back
- Asymmetry (unevenness) of the waist
- One shoulder blade being more noticeable than the other
- Chest shifted to one side
- Clothes fitting unevenly
- One hip being higher than the other
- Ribs more prominent on one side than the other

Figure 1.5.1 shows three of these common signs.

---

* A primary care provider may also be referred to as a general practitioner (GP).

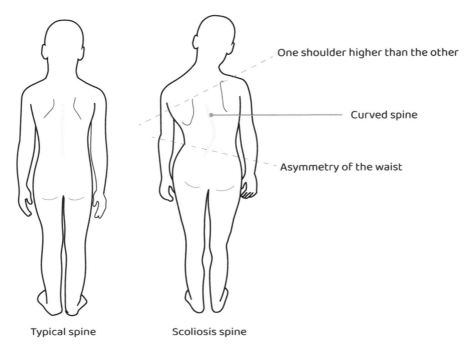

One shoulder higher than the other

Curved spine

Asymmetry of the waist

Typical spine   Scoliosis spine

Figure 1.5.1 Three common signs of scoliosis.

Primary care providers may routinely check for scoliosis during annual checkups.* The primary care provider may conduct an Adams forward bend test, which can help identify scoliosis by revealing asymmetry or signs of rotation and curvature of the spine. During this test, the individual bends forward and the provider examines the back from behind. As shown in Figure 1.5.2, when an individual with scoliosis bends over, one side may appear higher or more prominent than the other. If the primary care provider suspects scoliosis, they may have X-rays taken of the spine.

---

* In the US, children, adolescents, and adults are encouraged to visit their primary care provider every year.

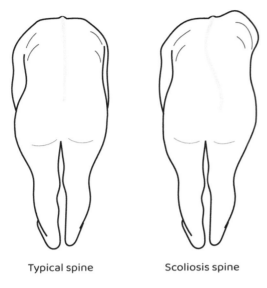

Typical spine   Scoliosis spine

Figure 1.5.2 Adams forward bend test

Children and adolescents who display signs and symptoms of scoliosis will be referred to a spine specialist. Their first visit may be with an orthopedic spine surgeon or an advanced practice provider (APP) such as a physician assistant (PA) or a nurse practitioner (NP).

Lila

The first time I remember hearing the term "scoliosis" was in a yearly checkup when I was about eight years old. My doctor told me they would need to keep an eye on it when things started getting worse. Until then, I had never even heard of scoliosis. I remember being confused because I felt fine and didn't know what the problem was with my back. I don't think I understood what it all meant until I was put in a back brace.

Tana

Lila was seven or eight years old when her pediatrician first mentioned that she could see a slight curvature in Lila's spine. This was during a routine check with Lila bending over and reaching toward her toes. The pediatrician said Lila may have idiopathic scoliosis, and we would need to continue to watch it.

At the time, I could tell that Lila didn't understand much of what the doctor was saying, but I still felt concerned, stressed, and disappointed for her, as she had already been through a fair amount of medical and health issues at a very young age, including previous surgery and diagnoses unrelated to her scoliosis. Even though it wouldn't have an immediate impact on Lila's life, it felt like yet one more health issue that would need to be monitored. In the first few months following this initial diagnosis, I was overly fixated on Lila's back and watched closely for any changes.

The next few years proved uneventful and unchanging. We went to Lila's appointments, our pediatrician would have her bend and reach for her toes, and then she would tell us that the curvature continued to remain slight and to check in again in a year. Because of this routine, I was lulled into thinking that medical intervention would not be necessary.

Lila was 12 when the pediatrician ordered an X-ray to get an idea of the significance of the curve. That made sense to me, given Lila's age and impending growth spurt, so I remained in my state of denial. But reality set in when the pediatrician called with the results, telling us that Lila had an S-curve that was measuring significantly more than she expected. She recommended we see a specialist as soon as possible. To be honest, I was hesitant, as Lila already had specialists at other children's hospitals in town.

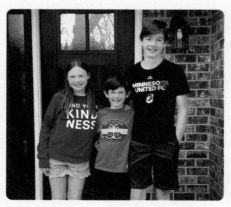

Lila (left) with her brothers, taken around the time of her diagnosis.

First appointment with a spine specialist

At the first visit to the spine specialist, there are many things they will ask about and observe. They will verify the presence of scoliosis through X-rays and a physical examination. After confirming scoliosis, the priority is to determine the cause. If there is no clear cause, it will be deemed idiopathic. The diagnosis of idiopathic scoliosis is not assigned until all other possible causes are ruled out. This is referred to as a "diagnosis of exclusion."

An individual's personal medical history, family medical history, physical exam, and imaging results are all puzzle pieces a spine specialist will use to learn more about the scoliosis and potential cause, and to then determine the best treatment plan.

a) Personal medical history

Taking a person's medical history, also called "past medical history," gives the spine specialist clues to possible causes and risk factors of the individual's scoliosis. This medical history includes the mother's experience during pregnancy as well as the individual's prior or current medical diagnoses, history of relevant symptoms such as missed developmental milestones, or previous medical procedures. It is possible that an individual, especially a young person, may present with scoliosis caused by a medical condition that has not yet been diagnosed.

b) Family medical history

Learning more about an individual's family medical history, including that of their parents, siblings, and grandparents, is an important part of the first appointment with a spine specialist. Certain types of scoliosis, or conditions that cause scoliosis, can have a genetic and heritable component, meaning they can run in families and can be passed down through generations.

c) Physical exam

The physical exam is another important piece of the puzzle when diagnosing scoliosis. During a physical exam, a spine specialist will conduct a nerve and skin exam and observe the individual walking, if they are able. The physical exam is a chance to look for signs of an underlying medical condition that may impact scoliosis care as well as overall health. The physical exam also offers the spine specialist a chance to learn more about the individual's scoliosis curve. Flexibility measurements may be performed, such as bending side to side, which can indicate the stiffness or flexibility of the curve. An Adams forward bend test can provide information about the amount of vertebral rotation and curvature. A scoliometer, a specifically designed level, can be used to measure the degree of vertebral rotation, as shown in Figure 1.5.3.

During the exam, the provider may also take photos of the individual to document asymmetry in the waistline or shoulder height. These initial photos and measurements record the baseline values and can be used to assess curve progression and the effectiveness of future treatment.

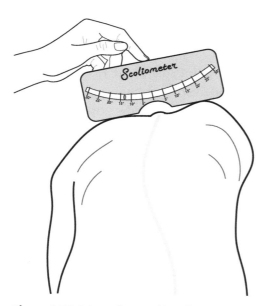

Figure 1.5.3 Adams forward bend test with a scoliometer to measure the degree of vertebral rotation.

d) Imaging results

X-ray imaging is a useful tool for diagnosing scoliosis. Full-length standing X-rays of the spine will be taken from the back and the side (Figure 1.5.4).

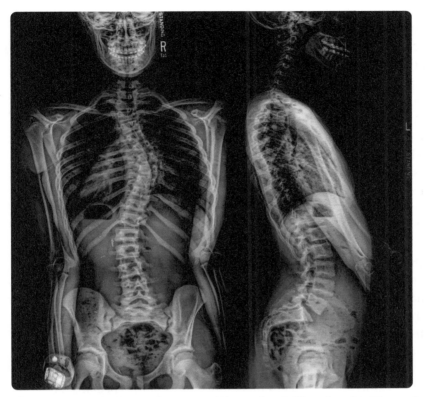

Figure 1.5.4 Scoliosis standing coronal X-ray view (left) and sagittal X-ray view (right).

These X-rays provide a two-dimensional view of the bones of the spine in the coronal and sagittal planes. At some hospitals and treatment centers, these standing films may be taken with technology that uses low-dose X-ray imaging and captures both the coronal and sagittal images at the same time. Associated software then allows for the production of two-dimensional images and a virtual three-dimensional reconstruction of the spine.

Spine X-rays are extremely important and useful for diagnosing scoliosis. On the coronal plane view, the spine of a person with scoliosis looks like an "S" or "C" instead of a straight line. The individual shown in Figure 1.5.4 has an S-shaped curve in their spine. **Note:** Throughout this book, the singular term "scoliosis curve" is used, but it is important to know that an individual may have more than one scoliosis curve.

Spine specialists measure the angle of the scoliosis curve on an X-ray in the coronal plane. This measurement is called a "Cobb angle" (also called the "curve magnitude"). It is determined by measuring the angle between the two most tilted vertebrae at the upper and lower ends of a spinal curve (Figure 1.5.5). The Cobb angle is the most commonly used measurement for quantifying the size of a spinal curve,[9] and it is the means by which a scoliosis diagnosis is made. Scoliosis is diagnosed when the Cobb angle is 10 degrees or greater. A slight curve of 1 to 9 degrees is called "spinal asymmetry" and is still considered typical (i.e., it is not considered scoliosis). The Cobb angle is measured on every X-ray over time to assess whether there is curve progression (increase in size).

Note that a very small difference of 1 degree in Cobb angle—from 9 to 10 degrees—changes the medical diagnosis from no scoliosis to scoliosis. Small differences in an individual's posture during the X-ray or who measures the Cobb angle can result in different angles. This is normal measurement variability, similar to when you take your body temperature three times with the same thermometer, getting three slightly different readings. Just as sequential temperature readings can vary, so can sequential Cobb angle measurements. It is typical for specialists to consider a scoliosis curve to have significantly progressed only if the change in Cobb angle is greater than 5 degrees. This is considered evidence of progression as opposed to measurement variability described above.

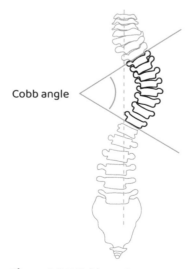

Cobb angle

Figure 1.5.5 Cobb angle measurement.

In addition to ordering a standing spine X-ray, the spine specialist may order a hand X-ray. The bones in the hand have important growth plates (areas of active, new bone growth that are made of cartilage and turn to solid bone when growing is done). The hand image allows the spine specialist to estimate how much skeletal growth remains for an individual.

After the initial spine visit, the spine specialist may also order a spine MRI, which provides detailed imaging of soft tissue (i.e., not bony) internal structures in the body, such as the spinal cord and intervertebral discs. A spine MRI can be used to check for any neural axis abnormalities, which are atypical findings within the brain or the spinal cord that affect 21 percent of individuals with idiopathic EOS.[10] Appendix 2 (online) addresses neural axis abnormalities.

Lila

I was 12 years old when I had my first appointment with a spine specialist for my back. I knew I had scoliosis, but I didn't know how severe it was. I had convinced myself that nothing was really wrong and nothing much would happen, so the talk about me getting a brace for my back and having to come to more appointments confused me and left me feeling like something was wrong with me or that I was too much of a hassle for the doctors and my family.

I wish I had been more prepared and had known that my scoliosis was worse than most of us thought. Initially, I felt a little scared and worried about what was going to happen to me.

The advice I have for others is to not feel ashamed that you have scoliosis and to not worry about people who are helping you: that's their job and they are happy to do what they can to make your back better. Also, as I learned, it's important to stay positive and just power through. As awful as the diagnosis may seem in the moment, things *will* get better.

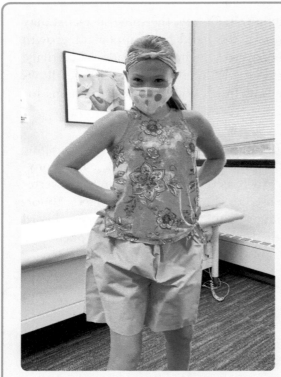

Lila at one of her first appointments with a spine specialist.

Key points Chapter 1

- The spine consists of vertebrae (bony structures with a hole for the spinal cord) and intervertebral discs (cartilage structures that sit between vertebral bodies).
- The spine protects the spinal cord, serves as an attachment point for the ribs and supporting muscles and ligaments, supports the weight of the body, and provides points of movement for the head and torso.
- Humans have 33 vertebrae, which are commonly grouped into five regions of the spine: cervical, thoracic, lumbar, sacral, and coccygeal.
- When looking at the side view of a person, the spine has distinct curvature. Lordosis is an inward curvature (arching toward the center of the body) and kyphosis is an outward curvature (rounding away from the center of the body).
- Typical spine curvature is a slight cervical lordosis, thoracic kyphosis, lumbar lordosis, and sacral kyphosis.
- Scoliosis is a condition in which there is an atypical three-dimensional curvature and rotation of the spine. The largest change from typical spine curvature occurs in the coronal plane.
- There are five types of scoliosis, classified by cause: idiopathic, congenital, neuromuscular, syndromic, and other.
- Idiopathic scoliosis is scoliosis that develops from an unknown cause. It is the most common type of scoliosis (affecting between 0.5 to 3.0 percent of the population).
- While diagnosis and treatment can be challenging, individuals with idiopathic scoliosis can expect to lead typical lives.
- Early-onset scoliosis (EOS) is scoliosis diagnosed prior to 10 years of age.
- The presence of scoliosis is verified by a spine specialist through X-ray images and a physical exam.
- The Cobb angle is the angle between the two most tilted vertebrae at the upper and lower ends of a spinal curve, as measured with X-ray images. Scoliosis is diagnosed when the Cobb angle on the coronal view is 10 degrees or greater.
- The diagnosis of idiopathic scoliosis is not assigned until all other possible causes are ruled out (diagnosis of exclusion).

Chapter 2

Idiopathic scoliosis

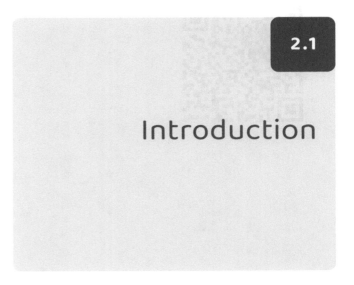

Introduction

> The pessimist complains about the wind;
> the optimist expects it to change;
> the realist adjusts the sails.
> **William Arthur Ward**

Idiopathic scoliosis is the most common form of scoliosis. Recall that idiopathic scoliosis develops with no definite cause, and that individuals with idiopathic scoliosis are otherwise typically developing with no related underlying medical condition.

The condition has a genetic component, as evidenced by the higher prevalence (6 to 11 percent) of adolescent idiopathic scoliosis in individuals who have first-degree family members with the same condition, but the exact genes involved remain unknown. In fact, there are likely many genes involved.[3] Additionally, twin studies show that identical twins are more likely to have scoliosis if one twin has scoliosis.[11] but the chance is less than 100 percent, which indicates that environmental factors that are not completely understood may be at play.

USEFUL WEB RESOURCES

Classification and related information

Science is the systematic classification of experience.
George Henry Lewes

Idiopathic scoliosis is classified based on age at diagnosis (Table 2.2.1). It may not be detected until years after it has begun to develop, so some spine specialists acknowledge that a 10-year-old diagnosed with a large curve, for example, likely has juvenile idiopathic scoliosis (JIS) rather than adolescent idiopathic scoliosis (AIS). As Table 2.2.1 shows, there are gender differences in the prevalence of idiopathic scoliosis within age groups. The reason for these gender differences is not known.

Curve characteristics, including the location and direction of the curve in the spine, also vary among individuals with idiopathic scoliosis. When a child or adolescent presents with curve characteristics that do not align with the typical curve characteristics as shown in Table 2.2.1, it may indicate that the scoliosis is nonidiopathic and will generally lead to further investigation to confirm the individual's diagnosis.

Table 2.2.1 Idiopathic scoliosis: classification, population demographics, and curve characteristics

CLASSIFICATION	AGE OF DIAGNOSIS	RELATIVE PREVALENCE	GENDER DIFFERENCES	CURVE CHARACTERISTICS
Infantile idiopathic scoliosis (IIS)	0 to 3 years	Least	More common in boys than girls	Left thoracic curve* Hypokyphosis in the thoracic region of the spine
Juvenile idiopathic scoliosis (JIS)	4 to 9 years		At the younger end of the age range, boys are diagnosed slightly more often. At the older end of the age range, girls are diagnosed slightly more often.	Right thoracic curve* Hypokyphosis in the thoracic region of the spine
Adolescent idiopathic scoliosis (AIS)	10 to 18 years	Most	At small curve sizes, males and females are diagnosed similarly.[12] As curve size increases, females are diagnosed much more often than males.[12]	Right thoracic curve*[3] Hypokyphosis in the thoracic region of the spine[3]

* A scoliosis curve can be described by the location and direction of the curve. A left thoracic curve is a scoliosis curve located in the thoracic region of the spine (see Figure 1.2.2) that curves to the left side of the body. A right thoracic curve is a scoliosis curve located in the thoracic region of the spine that curves to the right side of the body.

Risk factors

A risk factor is "any attribute, characteristic, or exposure of an individual that increases the likelihood of developing a disease or injury."[13] Having a first-degree family member* with idiopathic scoliosis is a risk factor for a child developing idiopathic scoliosis. Only some risk factors for idiopathic scoliosis are known; research continues to discover new information that will help better understand idiopathic scoliosis in the future.

Parents and children often wonder if there is anything they did to cause the scoliosis. The simple answer is no. While some family predispositions may increase the risk of idiopathic scoliosis, the following actions, which parents often ask about, are *not* linked to developing idiopathic scoliosis:

- Wearing a heavy backpack
- Having poor posture
- Either playing or not playing sports
- Sleeping in a certain position or on a certain mattress

---

* A parent, child, or full sibling.

Idiopathic scoliosis: Age of diagnosis

*Every star shines differently.
Don't compare your glow with anyone else's.
You shine and that's all that matters.*
Unknown

Classification of idiopathic scoliosis by age of diagnosis is important to understand, as it impacts the overall management philosophy of the individual's scoliosis. As age of diagnosis changes, characteristics such as body size, skeletal maturity, and overall risk of progression change. This section discusses idiopathic scoliosis at different ages.

Infantile idiopathic scoliosis

Infantile idiopathic scoliosis (IIS) is idiopathic scoliosis diagnosed in the first three years of life. The diagnosis of idiopathic scoliosis is not given until all other possible causes are ruled out. Especially in the case of IIS, the child will be closely watched for possible signs of an underlying condition, such as missed developmental milestones, to help determine if it is truly idiopathic scoliosis.

IIS can be classified as either resolving or progressive. It is common for IIS curves to resolve and straighten out naturally without treatment; this is known as spontaneous curve resolution. (Reported spontaneous curve resolution ranges from 12 to 92 percent).[14] This is the only form of idiopathic scoliosis that often resolves without treatment. However, some IIS curves will progress and eventually require treatment.

It is important for spine specialists to determine if the IIS curve is likely to resolve or progress so that children are not over- or undertreated. This risk assessment is often based on X-ray findings. Spine specialists examine the size of the curve, using the Cobb angle as well as the relationship between the vertebra furthest away from the center (the apical vertebra) (Figure 2.3.1) and the ribs attached on either side of it (Figures 2.3.2 and 2.3.3).

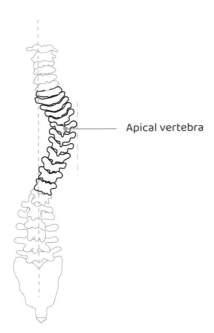

Apical vertebra

Figure 2.3.1 Apical vertebra (orange dashed line indicates the center of the body).

There are two measurements of the relative positions of the rib and vertebra that reveal the likelihood of curve progression in IIS:[15]

- **Rib phase:** The rib phase indicates the proximity of the rib to the apical vertebra on an X-ray. In phase 1, there is a gap between the rib and the apical vertebra. In phase 2, the rib appears to overlap the apical vertebra, indicating significant rotation of the spine (Figure 2.3.2).

- **Rib vertebral angle difference (RVAD):** RVAD indicates the difference in angles between the two ribs attached to the apical vertebra on an X-ray. RVAD is calculated by measuring the angle between each of the ribs attached to the apical vertebra. The difference between these two angles is then calculated (Figure 2.3.3). A larger angle difference indicates more significant rotation of the spine.

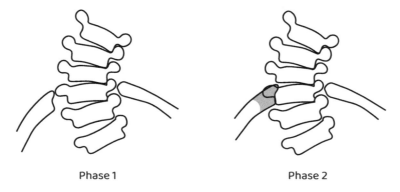

Phase 1   Phase 2

Figure 2.3.2 Rib phase.

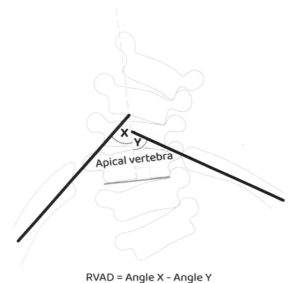

RVAD = Angle X - Angle Y

Figure 2.3.3 Rib vertebral angle difference (RVAD).

Transitioning from phase 1 ribs to phase 2 ribs is a sign of a progressive scoliosis curve.[15] Additionally, individuals with an RVAD of 20 degrees or greater are more likely to have a progressive scoliosis curve.[15] In contrast, individuals with an RVAD less than 20 degrees are far less likely to have a progressive scoliosis curve and more likely to experience spontaneous curve resolution.[15]

Juvenile idiopathic scoliosis

Juvenile idiopathic scoliosis (JIS) is idiopathic scoliosis diagnosed between the ages of four and nine years. Unlike IIS, JIS is not likely to spontaneously resolve without treatment; however, it can happen on rare occasions. One study reports resolution in 5 percent of individuals.[16]

JIS typically progresses steadily through early childhood but rapidly during the adolescent growth spurt.[16] Due to the presence of a scoliosis curve prior to the adolescent growth spurt, individuals with JIS are at higher risk of severe curve progression than those with adolescent idiopathic scoliosis.[17] Additionally, 20 percent of individuals with JIS have a neural axis abnormality (atypical structures within the brain and/or spinal cord),[17] so it is important for spine specialists to order an MRI to evaluate for this. See Appendix 2 (online).

Adolescent idiopathic scoliosis

Adolescent idiopathic scoliosis (AIS) is idiopathic scoliosis diagnosed between the ages of 10 to 18 years. Unlike the early-onset forms of idiopathic scoliosis (IIS and JIS), individuals with AIS have a lower likelihood of developing severe scoliosis since their curves develop later in life and thus have a shorter growth period for a curve to progress.[17] Some individuals with AIS may be diagnosed prior to their adolescent growth spurt, while others may be diagnosed when growth is complete (i.e., they are skeletally mature). Due to varying skeletal maturity in individuals with AIS, measurement tools for assessing how much growth an adolescent has remaining, such as the standardized skeletal maturity scoring systems addressed in section 2.4, are especially important. Large curves and/or curves in adolescents who are not yet skeletally mature are the most likely to continue to progress and require treatment.

Overview of treatment

Coming together is a beginning;
keeping together is progress;
working together is success.
Edward Everett Hale

There is currently no way to prevent idiopathic scoliosis, but there are many available treatment options. Though little may be known about the actual cause of idiopathic scoliosis, its treatment is well understood and studied. While the initial diagnosis and the treatment that follows may seem overwhelming, it is important to know that the outlook for most children and adolescents with idiopathic scoliosis is good. Idiopathic scoliosis is rarely life-threatening, and those who have it will usually lead a normal, healthy life with few limitations on physical function and activities, including sports.

Why treat idiopathic scoliosis?

Treatment can be time-consuming, costly, stressful, and unpleasant physically and emotionally for the individual and their family. So why treat idiopathic scoliosis in the first place?

Untreated scoliosis may progress and, if severe enough, can negatively affect those who have the condition through childhood and into adulthood. Treatment for idiopathic scoliosis focuses on *preventing curve progression* to keep the curve as small as possible as the child grows. The larger the curve, the greater the likelihood of continued curve progression[18] and for it to have a negative impact on the individual's health and quality of life. Often, the negative effects of untreated scoliosis, such as shortness of breath or back pain, are the result of scoliosis curve progression, and symptoms tend to worsen through adulthood. The main concerns with untreated, severe idiopathic scoliosis include adverse effects on cardiopulmonary (heart and lung) function, back pain, and psychosocial (psychological and social) challenges.

a) Cardiopulmonary function

Idiopathic scoliosis may impact the cardiopulmonary (heart and lung) function of some individuals. As well, individuals with idiopathic scoliosis curves greater than 80 degrees can have decreased heart function.[19]

Scoliosis can also impact lung function in two distinct ways.[20] First, the curving and rotating of the spine can limit the ability of the rib cage to expand and the lungs to fill with air, making it difficult to breathe or cough to clear the airways, especially during illness. Second, the limited space for the lungs prevents them from developing properly during growth. This is called restrictive lung disease. In typical development, chest growth occurs rapidly during the first five years of life,[21] and the development of alveoli, the air sacs in the lungs that allow for the exchange of oxygen and carbon dioxide, continues until eight years of age.[22] In a chest constricted by progressive scoliosis, the lungs do not continue to grow and develop, leading to an adult-sized body with the breathing capabilities of a small child.[20] This impact on the lungs, which indirectly affects the heart and the circulatory system, occurs on a spectrum of severity and is generally seen only in individuals with early-onset scoliosis (EOS) or with a curve size that exceeds 60 degrees.[18]

At their most severe, these effects are called "thoracic insufficiency syndrome" (TIS), defined as the inability of the thorax (spine, ribs, and sternum) to allow for normal breathing or lung growth.[20] TIS has been observed in idiopathic scoliosis.[23] Research shows little risk of TIS in individuals with idiopathic scoliosis that develops after age 10.[18,23] However, this group of individuals may still have a reduced lung capacity that causes shortness of breath and affects activities such as sports and exercise, depending on the size and location of their scoliosis curve.[18,24]

In summary, large, untreated scoliosis curves can negatively impact cardiopulmonary function in some individuals. This is a key reason why spine specialists recommend early treatment of scoliosis, especially in young children who are at risk of problems with cardiopulmonary function.

b) Back pain

One reason to treat scoliosis is to decrease the incidence and severity of back pain in adulthood. More adults with untreated adolescent idiopathic scoliosis experience chronic back pain than adults without scoliosis.[24] Because scoliosis disrupts the typical alignment of the body, the body adjusts to keep the head over the pelvis. This imbalance is believed to lead to increased reliance on the muscles required to stay upright, which is thought to lead to early muscle fatigue and pain in the back, buttocks, and thighs.[25] While this theory is held by many clinicians, it is as yet unproven.

c) Psychosocial challenges

Idiopathic scoliosis is commonly diagnosed during adolescence, a time that poses its own psychosocial challenges without the addition of a visible medical condition. Left untreated, having scoliosis can result in a negative self-image.[26,27] Individuals with adolescent idiopathic scoliosis report feeling embarrassed about their appearance, feeling inferior to peers, choosing to limit social interactions to avoid feeling different than peers, and wearing baggy clothes to hide their scoliosis.[28] An important part of the spine specialist's role when treating scoliosis is to try to address the nuances of individual experiences and provide support with the individual's best interest in mind.

Factors affecting treatment decisions

Research studies that follow individuals who have not had any intervention are called "natural history studies." Natural history studies suggest that idiopathic scoliosis treatment is necessary and that the timing of treatment is important for best outcomes. Early scoliosis treatment is important to:

- Prevent the need for surgical intervention: when a curve is smaller, nonsurgical treatment options are possible.
- Optimize growth and development: especially for individuals with EOS, it is important to prevent scoliosis progression to enable the chest and lungs to develop properly.
- Minimize surgical risks: individuals with smaller curves are less likely to experience surgical complications than individuals with larger curves.

As such, the foundation of all idiopathic scoliosis treatment is preventive in nature.

Not all treatment options are appropriate for every individual. Idiopathic scoliosis treatment recommendations are made by identifying size and location of the curve, age, and risk of the curve progressing.

Factors associated with idiopathic scoliosis curve progression include:

- **Curve size:** As the size of the curve increases, the risk of progression also increases.[18] Scoliosis curves greater than or equal to 50 degrees have the highest risk of progression.[18] Thus, a curve of 50 degrees or greater is typically the threshold for recommending surgical intervention because, at that curve size, it is believed that the benefits of surgery typically outweigh the risks.
- **Curve location:** Scoliosis curves located in the thoracic region of the spine have the highest risk of progression.[18]
- **Skeletal maturity:** Children and adolescents who are still growing (skeletally immature) are more likely to have progression of their scoliosis curves than adolescents who are near the end of their growth (skeletally mature).[29]

- **Early adolescence:** Early adolescence is associated with an accelera-
  tion in the rate of growth, which is associated with an increased rate
  of curve progression.[30]

Spine specialists have many tools to assess the risk of curve progression.
Curve size and curve location can be identified through X-ray imaging
and physical exam. Growth remaining is assessed through a combination of factors, none of which provide a perfect answer. However,
when used in combination, these factors provide spine specialists with
an estimate of growth remaining. These factors include:

- **Age:** Age provides an estimate of how much growth remains.
- **Height tracking:** Examining change in height over time (rate of
  growth) allows spine specialists to determine if the individual
  has entered their adolescent growth spurt, a time of rapid growth
  and scoliosis curve progression, or if they have yet to begin this
  growth spurt.
- **Signs of puberty:** Physical examination assessing for signs of puberty,
  such as the development of breasts or pubic hair, are helpful for
  determining how much growth an individual has left. On average,
  boys reach their adult height three and a half years after the first
  signs of puberty.[31] Spine specialists also track the onset of a young
  girl's first period. Typically, girls reach their adult height two and a
  half to three years after they get their first period.[31]
- **Skeletal maturity:** Spine specialists use X-ray imaging of the hand,
  pelvis, or upper arm to track the "bone age" of an individual.
  These bones are commonly included in spine X-rays and are easy
  to track over time. When growing, bones have growth plates that
  are "open." (Growth plates are areas of active, new bone growth
  that are made of cartilage and turn to solid bone when growth is
  complete.) Because X-rays do not detect soft tissue such as cartilage,
  open growth plates look like gaps in the bones on an X-ray. Open
  growth plates tell spine specialists that there is still growth remaining. As an individual becomes more skeletally mature, their growth
  plates close—the cartilage fills in with bone. The order of closure
  has led to the development of a standardized scoring system that
  helps to determine an individual's skeletal maturity. Standardized
  skeletal maturity scoring systems are detailed below and shown in
  Figure 2.4.1:

○ **Triradiate cartilage**—growth plates in the hip joint. Scoring is either "open," which indicates skeletal immaturity or "closed," which indicates being more skeletally mature.

○ **Risser sign**—a growth plate that forms across the top of each side of the pelvis. Scoring is from 0 to 5, with 0 being the most skeletally immature and 5 being skeletally mature.

○ **Proximal Humerus Ossification System (PHOS)**—a growth plate in the upper arm bone. Scoring is from 1 to 5, with 1 being the most skeletally immature and 5 being skeletally mature.

○ **Sanders stage**—growth plates in the bones of the hand and wrist. Scoring is from 1 to 8, with 1 being the most skeletally immature and 8 being skeletally mature. The score of 7 is divided into 7a and 7b, based on partial closure versus complete closure of the ulna (long bone in the arm) growth plate.

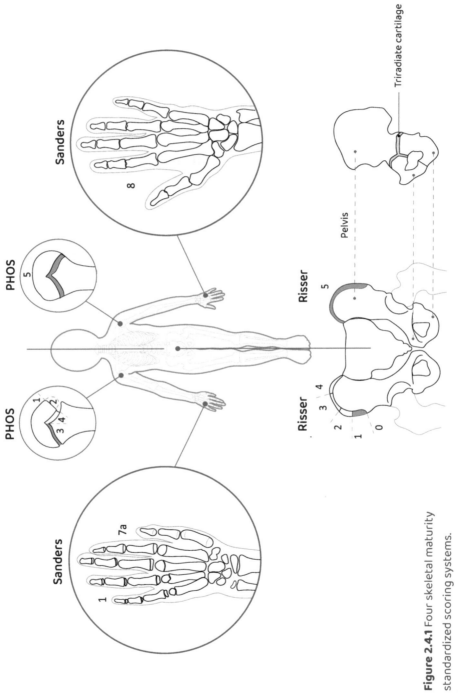

Figure 2.4.1 Four skeletal maturity standardized scoring systems.

There are many nuances to treatment recommendations. In addition to identifying the risk of curve progression, it is also important to consider the unique needs of the individual. The suggested treatment should be feasible for families to adhere to and match the individual's goals for function and quality of life. Decisions can be made using a shared decision-making model that includes the perspectives of the spine specialist and the individual and their family.

An overview of treatment options follows. Specific treatment indications and management strategies are addressed in Chapter 3.

Overview of treatment options and goals

Treatment options for scoliosis can range from nonsurgical methods, such as observation with repeat X-rays, to surgical methods, such as spinal fusion. Treatment options include the following (note that goals are shown in italics):

- **Observation:** Regular spine X-rays and clinical exams with a spine specialist *to monitor scoliosis curve for possible progression.*
- **Bracing:** A spinal brace that applies corrective forces to the spine *to slow or stop scoliosis curve progression.*
- **Casting:** A full-torso cast (hardened plaster or fiberglass that must be cut off to remove) that applies corrective forces to the spine *to improve the scoliosis curve (decrease the Cobb angle) or slow or stop scoliosis curve progression.*
- **Surgery:** Surgery performed *to prevent future progression and improve the scoliosis curve (decrease the Cobb angle).* There are many types of scoliosis surgery. The most common type is spinal fusion, defined as fusing (joining together) two or more vertebrae in the spine; screws and metal rods are typically used to hold the spine in the straightened position and facilitate fusion between bones.

These treatment options are shown in Figure 2.4.2.

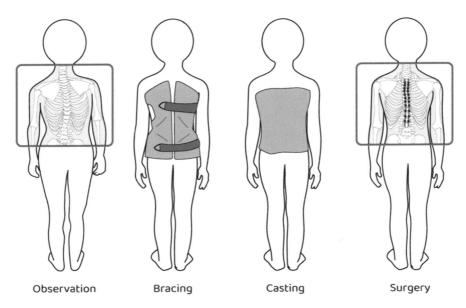

| Observation | Bracing | Casting | Surgery |

Figure 2.4.2 Four treatment options for idiopathic scoliosis.

As the child grows, the scoliosis progression may slow or increase, resulting in treatment plans changing. It is common for an individual to undergo multiple treatment types over the course of their childhood and adolescence. For example, an individual may be observed for a period of time, then prescribed bracing treatment if their curve progresses.

The appropriate treatment chosen and the related goals depend primarily on individual patient goals and specific surgical indications. Indications include, but are not limited to, size of the curve, risk of curve progression, and skeletal maturity of the child. A summary of the current indications and goals of treatment for scoliosis at Gillette Children's is given in Table 2.4.1. Treatment indications and goals may vary at other hospitals and treatment centers. Surgical guidelines are general and depend on the surgery type (see Chapter 4 for surgery types). Clinical practice continually evolves.

It is important to note that for *most* individuals, scoliosis cannot be "cured" (i.e., to achieve a Cobb angle less than 10 degrees). For some children with IIS, their curve may spontaneously resolve, or casting treatment can reduce the curve to less than 10 degrees, but that is the exception. The more common outcome and realistic goal is to have a small enough residual curve after treatment that will not adversely affect quality of life.

Tana

Lila first met with the spine specialist shortly after she turned 12, the summer before she was starting middle school and during COVID restrictions. During that appointment, he told Lila she would need to be fitted for a brace to wear during the day. I could see Lila getting emotional behind her mask and tears welling up in her eyes. She held it together just long enough to get back to our car. Before I could say anything, she looked at me and asked, "Why is there so much wrong with me?" I instinctively responded, "There is so much that is right with you." And I meant it. I mention this because I think it set the tone for the months and years to come on Lila's scoliosis journey. Since then, while I'm certain she has had difficult feelings and thoughts, I have never heard Lila ask, "Why me?" Instead, she has faced every stage of her scoliosis with appreciation and determination.

As soon as we were home from that appointment, I immediately started researching types of scoliosis braces on the Internet. I think I was also hoping to find that the scoliosis brace that I knew kids were wearing 30 years ago had been reinvented. I saw some braces online that looked like sports bras, and secretly hoped this was all Lila would need to wear. I didn't share any of this information with Lila.

We also told Lila's brothers about her having to wear a brace, explaining what it was and why and when she would need to wear it. As a family, we agreed that we would support Lila any way we could, and that this was Lila's information to share with whomever she was comfortable sharing it with. We consistently reminded Lila that her wearing a brace did not affect who she is in any way.

> ## Lila
>
> At my first appointment, the doctor suggested a back brace for me that I would wear 18 hours a day. This was a shock to me as I hadn't really known what to expect at this appointment. I finally started to understand what my scoliosis treatment might look like when the doctor showed me a sample brace, explaining how I would put it on using the Velcro straps on the back and sliding my body through a small gap in the side, pointing out the padding in the sides.
>
> The orthotist took some measurements of my back and explained the interesting shape and what the cutouts in the brace design were for. I felt very emotional about it all and I was very opposed to the idea of wearing a brace; I didn't want to talk about it anymore. My mom was with me at that appointment, and afterwards, we sat in the car and cried for a while. Everything that had been worrying me felt better as I cried, and my mom tried to help me understand a little more about the bracing.

Overall IIS management philosophy

Based on the current Cobb angle, rib phase, RVAD measurements, and observed changes with time, spine specialists determine if the curve is progressing or resolving. If it is resolving, observation is recommended with appropriate follow-up X-rays. For curves that are progressing, the best treatment plan will be recommended. This treatment recommendation may change over time depending on the amount of curve progression the child experiences, the assessed risk of further progression, and the response to treatment.

Often, with small scoliosis curves, the best treatment is observation. Children with IIS have a large amount of "growth potential," meaning they will experience a lot of skeletal growth during their first three years of life. Because skeletal growth is closely related to scoliosis curve progression, spine specialists will want to closely monitor a child as they grow to prevent rapid curve progression. If the scoliosis curve progresses during observation, further treatment options will be considered. At this stage, it is typical to recommend nonsurgical treatment such as wearing a brace or cast to stabilize or correct the scoliosis curve. Surgical treatment is highly unlikely during the first three years of life.

Overall JIS management philosophy

Most children with JIS require treatment for their scoliosis.[17] However, observation may be appropriate in individuals who have a small scoliosis curve (less than 20 degrees) at diagnosis. If the scoliosis curve progresses, the recommendation is often to begin wearing a brace to either prevent further progression and avoid surgery, or to slow the progression enough to delay surgery. Surgical options for individuals with EOS can carry risks and high complication rates.[14] Therefore, spine specialists often hope to delay surgery in children with JIS to allow the child to reach an appropriate level of thoracic growth (chest height and width), in turn allowing their lungs to continue developing prior to surgical treatment. For individuals who experience curve progression despite brace treatment, surgery will be recommended once deemed necessary.

Overall AIS management philosophy

As opposed to identifying if the curve is progressive or resolving (as with IIS) or evaluating if the individual has reached an appropriate level of thoracic growth (as with JIS), most treatment decisions for AIS are made based on the individual's current curve size and their level of skeletal maturity. At this age, individuals have typically grown to a point that chest and lung size are no longer a concern as they are in JIS. Instead, general risk of scoliosis curve progression (based on curve size and skeletal maturity) will guide treatment recommendations.

For example, skeletally immature (still growing) individuals with a small- to moderate-size curve can wear a brace to slow or stop progression and reduce the likelihood of surgery.[32,33,34,35] In contrast, bracing is not an appropriate treatment option for individuals who are skeletally mature (almost finished or finished growing). Similarly, for surgery, a skeletally immature individual with a 45-degree curve may be considered appropriate for surgical intervention due to their likelihood of continued growth and curve progression. In contrast, surgery may not be considered to treat a 45-degree curve in an adolescent nearing skeletal maturity because they are at lower risk of continued progression.

Table 2.4.1 Treatment options, indications, and goals for idiopathic scoliosis at Gillette Children's

TREATMENT OPTIONS	INDICATIONS	GOALS
Observation		
IIS	Cobb angle less than 20 degrees	Monitor scoliosis curve through repeat X-ray images for possible progression
JIS	Cobb angle less than 20 degrees	
AIS (skeletally immature)	Cobb angle less than 20 degrees	
AIS (skeletally mature)	Cobb angle between 30 and 50 degrees	
Bracing		
IIS	Cobb angle 20 to 45 degrees AND either: • RVAD greater than 20 degrees OR • Rib phase 2	Slow or stop scoliosis curve progression Prevent or delay surgery
JIS	Cobb angle between 20 and 45 degrees	
AIS (skeletally immature)	Cobb angle between 20 and 45 degrees	
AIS (skeletally mature)	Not an appropriate treatment once skeletally mature	
Casting		
IIS	All the following: • Age 1 to 3 years • Cobb angle greater than 20 degrees • RVAD greater than 20 degrees OR rib phase 2	Slow or stop curve progression Improve the scoliosis curve (decrease the Cobb angle) Prevent or delay surgery

Cont'd.

TREATMENT OPTIONS	INDICATIONS	GOALS
Casting		
JIS	Not typically recommended for individuals older than 3 years.	
AIS (skeletally immature)	Not typically initiated for individuals older than 3 years.	
AIS (skeletally mature)	Not typically initiated for individuals older than 3 years.	
Surgery		
IIS	Unlikely during the first three years of life; only considered if the scoliosis continues to progress and has a negative impact on the child's health and quality of life	Stop curve progression Improve the scoliosis curve (decrease the Cobb angle)
JIS	Cobb angle greater than or equal to 40 to 50 degrees, depending on surgery type and level of skeletal maturity OR if the scoliosis continues to progress and has a negative impact on the child's health and quality of life	Allow continued spinal growth
AIS (skeletally immature)	Cobb angle greater than or equal to 40 to 50 degrees, depending on surgery type and level of skeletal maturity.	Stop curve progression Improve the spinal curve (decrease the Cobb angle)
AIS (skeletally mature)	Cobb angle greater than 50 degrees	Achieve a balanced spine and posture

Evidence-based medicine and shared decision-making

Evidence-based medicine (or evidence-based practice) is "the conscientious, explicit, and judicious use of current best evidence in making decisions about the care of individual patients."[36] It combines the best available external clinical evidence from research with the clinical expertise of the professional.[36] Family priorities and preferences are also considered.[37]

Since clinical expertise can vary, it is important to know that recommendations in this book may vary among hospitals and treatment centers. Furthermore, treatment is not "one size fits all"; it must be customized. The best practice for managing idiopathic scoliosis is to have a multidisciplinary care team skilled in providing scoliosis care and engaging with a family in a shared decision-making model—a process in which the family is actively involved in making decisions about medical treatment and care. The child's involvement in this process will vary depending on their age and developmental level. The key to shared decision-making is communicating and incorporating the principles of evidence-based medicine.[38]

The following, in alphabetical order, lists individuals on the multidisciplinary spine team. This list is not exhaustive, and not all teams will have representation from the same disciplines. Team members may have different titles, and roles may vary in different countries:

- Advanced practice provider (nurse practitioner or physician assistant)
- Anesthesiologist and nurse anesthetist (administration of medication resulting in sleep-like state needed for surgery)
- Case manager
- Child life specialist (child development and effective coping through play)
- Neurosurgeon
- Nurse
- Nutrition specialist
- Orthotist (brace specialist)
- Pediatrician and critical care provider
- Physical therapist
- Pulmonologist (lungs and airway)
- Psychologist
- Respiratory therapist
- Social worker
- Spine surgeon

Key points Chapter 2

- Individuals with a first-degree family member with idiopathic scoliosis have a higher chance of developing it.
- Idiopathic scoliosis is classified based on age at diagnosis—infantile (0 to 3 years), juvenile (4 to 9 years) and adolescent (10 to 18 years).
- It is common for infantile idiopathic scoliosis (IIS) to resolve and straighten out naturally without treatment, whereas this is rare for juvenile idiopathic scoliosis (JIS) and adolescent idiopathic scoliosis (AIS).
- Due to the presence of a scoliosis curve prior to the adolescent growth spurt, individuals with JIS are at higher risk of severe curve progression than those with AIS.
- The general treatment philosophy for idiopathic scoliosis focuses on preventing curve progression. The larger the curve, the greater the likelihood of continued progression and for it to have a negative impact on the individual's health and quality of life.
- The main concerns with untreated severe idiopathic scoliosis include cardiopulmonary function, back pain, and psychosocial (psychological and social) challenges.
- Early scoliosis treatment is important to prevent surgical intervention, optimize growth and development, and minimize surgical risks.
- Spine specialists use several factors to estimate how much growth a child has remaining: age, height tracking, signs of puberty, and skeletal maturity (using X-ray images of the hand, pelvis, or upper arm).
- Scoliosis treatment options include observation, bracing, casting, or surgery. It is common for an individual to undergo multiple treatment types.
- If children with IIS experience curve progression, it is typical to recommend nonsurgical treatment such as wearing a brace or cast.
- Most children with JIS require treatment. Spine specialists often aim to delay surgery in children with JIS to allow the child to reach an appropriate thoracic growth for optimal cardiopulmonary function prior to surgery.
- The best practice for managing idiopathic scoliosis is to have a care team skilled in providing scoliosis care engaging with a family in a shared decision-making model.

Chapter 3

Nonsurgical treatment

Introduction

The price of success is hard work, dedication to the job at hand,
and the determination that whether we win or lose,
we have applied the best of ourselves to the task at hand.

Vince Lombardi

Nonsurgical treatment of scoliosis, also referred to as nonoperative or conservative treatment, is treatment that does not require surgery. Nonsurgical treatments addressed in this chapter include observation, bracing, casting, physical therapy, and alternative and complementary treatments (see Table 3.1.1).

Table 3.1.1 Nonsurgical treatment of scoliosis

TREATMENT	EXPLANATION OF TREATMENT
Observation	Regular spine X-rays and clinical exams with a spine specialist to monitor scoliosis curve progression
Bracing	A spinal orthosis (removable brace) that applies corrective forces to the spine to slow or stop scoliosis curve progression
Casting	A full-torso cast (hardened plaster or fiberglass that must be removed by a clinician) that applies corrective forces to the spine to reduce the scoliosis curve size or stop/slow scoliosis curve progression; also used to improve balance and alignment of the torso
Physical therapy scoliosis-specific exercises (PSSE)	Exercise sessions with a specially trained physical therapist; involves stretching, strengthening, postural corrections, breathing techniques, and education to help the individual control their posture independently
Vitamin D_3 and calcium supplements	Daily vitamin D_3 and calcium supplements to help with low bone density in individuals with idiopathic scoliosis and that may slow scoliosis curve progression[39,40]

The overall goal of nonsurgical treatment is to slow or stop curve progression to prevent or delay surgery. Thus, early intervention with nonsurgical treatment is encouraged to optimize outcomes and maximize an individual's chance of avoiding future surgery. The decision of which and when nonsurgical treatments are appropriate is shared between the family and medical care provider.

USEFUL WEB RESOURCES

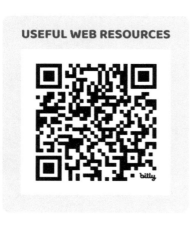

Observation

How poor are they that have not patience!
What wound did ever heal but by degrees?
William Shakespeare

Observation management of scoliosis requires regular X-rays and clinical exams with a spine specialist. Observation is generally recommended for individuals with a Cobb angle less than 20 degrees and some larger curves in skeletally mature individuals. Candidates for observation are deemed to have a low risk of scoliosis curve progression; thus, treatments such as bracing or surgery may not be necessary for their scoliosis, or at least not yet.

The goal of observation is to monitor any progression of the scoliosis curves through repeat X-rays and clinical exams. True curve progression is considered if there is a change in Cobb angle greater than 5 degrees. Repeat X-rays and clinical exams are typically scheduled every four to six months for skeletally immature individuals. This may extend to 6 to

12 months for individuals who are close to skeletal maturity or longer for those who have reached skeletal maturity.*

During each visit with a spine specialist, the child will have new X-rays taken of their spine, and possibly of their hand to measure remaining skeletal growth. The spine specialist will also obtain height and weight measurements and perform a physical exam. If the scoliosis curve progresses and seems likely to continue progressing, other treatment options will be discussed.

---

* A follow-up schedule for adults (skeletally mature) with idiopathic scoliosis is discussed in section 5.2.

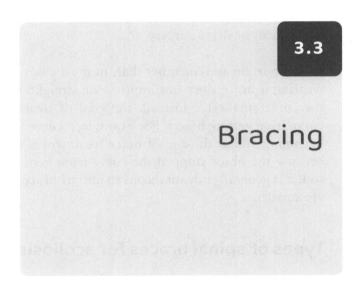

3.3

Bracing

Opportunities do not come with their values stamped upon them.
Waltbie Davenport Babcock

Wearing a spinal orthosis, also referred to as a brace, is the most common nonsurgical treatment for progressive scoliosis curves. The term "orthosis" comes from the Greek word "ortho," which means "to straighten or align." A spinal brace is designed to provide support and improve alignment of the spine by applying specific pressures to the torso to slow or stop the curve from progressing.

The Scoliosis Research Society (SRS) recommends brace treatment for individuals who have curves measuring 25 to 45 degrees and are skeletally immature.[41] However, this Cobb angle range may vary slightly depending on the treating spine specialist and typical bracing practices at the medical center. For example, individuals with a Cobb angle less than 25 degrees are commonly braced at Gillette Children's if they are at high risk for progressing, such as in cases where there is a family history of scoliosis or the individual presents at a young age and is already showing rapid curve progression.

Goals for bracing are to:

- Slow or stop curve progression
- Prevent or delay surgery

It is important to remember that, in most cases of idiopathic scoliosis, wearing a brace does not improve or straighten the curve (i.e., make the curve smaller).[42] Instead, the goal of treatment is to prevent the curve from getting bigger. For example, a curve that is 35 degrees at the beginning and at the end of brace treatment is considered a "success" because the brace stopped the curve from getting bigger. For this reason, it is generally advantageous to initiate brace treatment when curves are smaller.

Types of spinal braces for scoliosis

There are several types of spinal braces used to treat scoliosis. Each is named for the region of the spine they impact. The most common type of spinal brace is the thoraco-lumbo-sacral orthosis (TLSO), which is the focus of this section (see Table 3.3.1).

A TLSO is typically made from molded, rigid plastic that extends from the armpits to the pelvis, not limiting hip motion. Scoliosis TLSOs are custom made for the individual to provide the best comfort and scoliosis curve control. A TLSO may be fabricated at the medical care center or at a company that specializes in making them. Once the TLSO is made, it is fit to the child by the orthotist.*

Scoliosis TLSOs can vary in the design, the type of padding, and material choice (type of plastic); however, regardless of the details, the TLSO must be fitted well and designed appropriately for the individual's specific curve characteristics. Prolonged and specialized expert training is necessary for the orthotist to make a well-fitting, effective brace.

---

* An orthotist is a health care professional who designs and fits orthoses (braces) working in conjunction with a spine specialist who provides the prescription. The two must communicate well and work together as a team.

The two types are full-time and nighttime hypercorrective TLSOs. A full-time TLSO is prescribed to be worn during the day and night, typically 18 to 23 hours per day. It should be removed for physical activity such as sports, physical therapy, and workouts.

A nighttime hypercorrective TLSO is prescribed to be worn only while lying down, typically when an individual is sleeping. The nighttime hypercorrective TLSO takes advantage of the elimination of gravity. When lying down, the spine is more correctible, and greater corrective forces can comfortably be applied to the scoliosis curve—hence the term "hypercorrective."

Table 3.3.1 Types of spinal braces for scoliosis

TYPE	CURVE LOCATION	WEAR TIME	IMAGE
Full-time thoraco-lumbo-sacral orthosis (TLSO)	Primary curve in the thoracic and lumbar spine	18 to 23 hours a day (worn day and night)	
Nighttime hypercorrective thoraco-lumbo-sacral orthosis (TLSO)	Primary curve in the thoracic and lumbar spine	8 to 12 hours a day (worn at night only)	

Full-time versus nighttime hypercorrective TLSO treatment

Depending on the curve size and the amount of growth potential an individual has, the spine specialist may recommend that the brace be worn full-time (day and night) or only at night.

Full-time TLSO treatment is considered the "gold standard," meaning that treatment with this type of brace is most supported by research and has been shown to be effective at slowing or stopping curve progression and preventing surgery when worn for the prescribed amount of time.[32,33,34,35]

In comparison, high-quality research on the use of a nighttime hypercorrective TLSO is limited and more research is needed to determine its efficacy in treating individuals with adolescent idiopathic scoliosis (AIS).[43] However, the research that does exist suggests that treatment with a nighttime hypercorrective TLSO may be comparable to treatment with a full-time TLSO for individuals with idiopathic curves in the thoracolumbar* or lumbar region of the spine and those who are more skeletally mature when they start wearing a brace (Risser sign of 1 or 2 rather than Risser 0).[43]

Starting brace treatment

Once the spine specialist recommends brace treatment, the individual will be referred to an orthotist who specializes in designing and fitting spinal braces.

The first step is to have an evaluation with the orthotist. The orthotist will gather information about the individual and their specific scoliosis curve, including how flexible the curve is and the individual's overall posture and balance. The orthotist will measure the individual's body and capture the shape of their torso with a plaster mold (a wrap with smooth paste that hardens when it dries) or digital scanning technology. The orthotist will then design the brace (in consultation with

---

* A thoracolumbar scoliosis curve is located where the lower thoracic region and upper lumbar region of the spine meet.

the spine specialist) according to the individual's X-rays and physical exam; in other words, it will be customized for the person being treated. Individuals may also choose a color or pattern for their brace.

The second step is the brace fitting. During this appointment, the orthotist fits the brace, customizing the plastic and padding as appropriate for the scoliosis curve while making sure that the individual is comfortable wearing it. The orthotist will teach the individual and parent how to put the brace on and how tight to pull the straps. They will check the pressure on the skin throughout the fitting appointment to be sure no parts of the brace could cause discomfort or breakdown of the skin. They will give instructions on how to get used to wearing the brace (called the "break-in"), how to care for and monitor skin integrity, and when to follow up. It is important for the orthotist to regularly check the brace fit and function as the individual grows.

The brace-fitting appointment is an important time for the individual and parent to voice any concerns they have about the fit and comfort. The orthotist is a valuable resource and can help individuals figure out ways to integrate the brace into home and school life.

An X-ray of the individual wearing their brace, called an "in-brace X-ray" is taken to check that all components of the brace are applying forces appropriately to the spine. The in-brace X-ray is done either at the brace-fitting appointment or at a clinic appointment shortly after. The individual's spine may look straighter or "corrected" in this X-ray because of the external forces that the brace is applying; however, once the brace is removed, the spine most likely will return to its pre-brace position. This is because braces help slow or stop curve progression, not improve or straighten the curve.

Lila

At the appointment when I was actually fit for my daytime brace, I remember my orthotist making a mold for the fit, and then I had to take it on and off several times so they could make small adjustments for my comfort. While we waited for each adjustment, my mom and I would visit the café for a snack and pass the time playing cards. It was a very long and tiring day.

Tana

Lila's first brace-fitting appointment was set within a few weeks at Gillette Children's in downtown Saint Paul, Minnesota. I didn't know it then, but over the next 18 months, we would spend a lot of time with our orthotist.

Two memories stick out about that first fitting appointment. The first was seeing the hard, plastic-looking, torso-length scoliosis braces hanging up in the room. They looked unforgiving, and I could imagine that to Lila they looked uncomfortable and scary, not at all like a sports bra. I understood that the purpose of this brace was essentially to guide Lila's body, but seeing it there was undoubtedly the most difficult part of the appointment.

The second thing I remember about that appointment was Lila putting on a tight slip-like cloth dress and watching the orthotist apply a plaster-like substance over her body. I think he also took some photos, and then Lila looked through the catalog of color and print options for the brace. That was the easy part. Lila loves color, but she decided that she wanted to only tell her friends about her brace and try to conceal it from others in school as much as possible, so she selected the tan color.

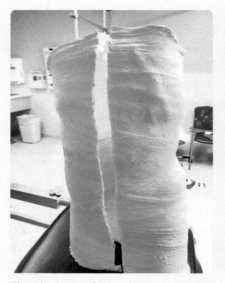 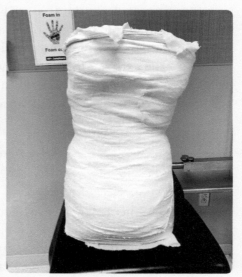

The plaster mold used to capture the shape of Lila's torso at her first appointment with an orthotist. This plaster mold was used to create her brace.

Within a week or two, we were back to pick up Lila's custom-made daytime brace. The orthotist handed her a seamless shirt to put on first and then showed her how to put the brace on over that. That was a learning experience; I remember the perplexed look on Lila's face. The brace had about a 1-inch (2.5 cm) opening in the back from the top to the bottom. Lila had to use all her strength to manipulate herself sideways into the brace through that opening, and as she was squeezing in, twist the brace so that the opening was in the back. The brace covered her entire torso and tucked under her armpits. It had two straps, one near her upper back and one near her lower back. There was a hole cut out in the front of the brace for her chest, but other than that, her entire torso was covered.

We had been told the brace-fitting process would take hours, and it did. I think we were at the hospital for five or six hours that day. It was a repetitive process of trying it on, the orthotist looking for areas of rubbing and asking Lila questions about comfort, then making markings to help shape and mold or cut off parts that rubbed. During the time the orthotist was adjusting the brace, Lila and I would go to the coffee shop for a break to get a snack or drink. We talked a lot during that time about the brace and how it might affect her every day, but I tried to let Lila lead the conversation so as to not overwhelm her. Those "breaks" were also a good opportunity to think through questions we had for the orthotist.

Duration of brace treatment

The duration of brace treatment depends mostly on skeletal maturity but can also depend on other factors such as age, curve size, and curve progression. If the curve remains under surgical magnitude (typically less than 50 degrees but may be 40 to 50 degrees depending on the individual's level of skeletal maturity), bracing will continue until growth is finished. That means that for individuals who start bracing when they are young (e.g., less than five years old) and have a significant amount of growth left, brace treatment may last for many years. More commonly, the total time of bracing is much shorter (18 to 24 months).

Throughout brace treatment, the individual will have regular clinic visits with the spine specialist and the orthotist. A brace generally needs to be adjusted by the orthotist every 3 to 6 months to accommodate growth, and it usually needs to be replaced every 12 to 18 months.

Ending brace treatment

For individuals who have been wearing a full-time TLSO, the spine specialist may begin a brace "wean" when the individual's growth starts to slow down. This means the wear time is slowly reduced over a period of 6 to 12 months as the individual approaches skeletal maturity. Research supports starting this weaning process when an individual reaches a Sanders stage 7b (see section 2.4).[44] An example of a wean schedule is reducing wear time from 18 to 23 hours per day to 12 hours per day for six months, and then reducing to 8 to 10 hours of wear (which typically means nighttime wear) for another six months. Note that nighttime wear is the final step in weaning before the brace is discontinued. For individuals being treated with a nighttime hypercorrective TLSO, a wean is often not required and they are simply instructed to stop brace wear once they reach skeletal maturity.

Brace treatment may end before skeletal maturity if a curve has progressed to a size that requires surgery (typically recommended at a Cobb angle of 50 degrees but may be 40 to 50 degrees depending on the individual's level of skeletal maturity).

Brace efficacy

In individuals with idiopathic scoliosis, two outcomes commonly used to measure bracing success are:[45]

- Five degrees or less of curve progression during brace treatment
- Avoiding surgery (typically meaning that the Cobb angle does not progress to 50 degrees or more)

When a scoliosis curve progresses 6 degrees or more during brace treatment, or if surgery is recommended due to curve progression beyond 50 degrees, this may be called "treatment failure." Successful bracing treatment in AIS is correlated with wear time.[32,33,34,35] In a landmark multicenter, randomized controlled trial, two groups of individuals with AIS were studied: a full-time brace treatment group and an observation group that did not wear a brace.[32] The brace treatment group was successful in preventing progression to 50 degrees 75 percent of the time compared to the observation group, which was successful only 42 percent of the time. Adolescents who wore the brace for more hours had a greater chance of success with brace treatment.

Although wear time is extremely important, the risk of treatment failure is not equal for all individuals with AIS, even with perfect adherence to the prescribed wear time. The following full-time brace failure risk factors have been identified for individuals with AIS: [34,35,46,47]

- Poor adherence to prescribed full-time wear (less than 10 to 13 hours per day).
- Significant amount of growth remaining at the start of brace treatment (Risser 0, triradiate cartilage open). For example, individuals with open triradiate cartilage at baseline have a 30 percent *greater* risk of treatment failure than those with closed triradiate cartilage at baseline.
- Cobb angle greater than or equal to 40 degrees prior to reaching adolescent growth spurt. For example, individuals with a 40-degree curve at baseline had a 40 percent *greater* risk of treatment failure than individuals with a 25-degree curve at baseline.
- Poor correction of the scoliosis curve in the brace as seen on the first in-brace X-ray.
- Large amount of vertebral rotation (rotation of the spine in the axial plane).
- Curves in the thoracic region.
- Osteopenia (a lower bone density than is typical for the individual's age in the general population).
- Higher body mass index (BMI), which can make it difficult to achieve adequate brace fit and in-brace curve correction.

Knowing these risk factors, spine specialists choose appropriate candidates for brace treatment, meaning those who are most likely to benefit from wearing the brace. Clinical tools, such as a risk calculator,* can guide spine specialists, orthotists, individuals and their families in being able to assess the risk of progression by using their baseline characteristics. Together, they can decide if treatment with a brace is likely to be beneficial and therefore warranted.[34,48]

Bracing challenges

While bracing has been shown to be an effective treatment method for scoliosis and can prevent the need for surgery, it can also be challenging for the individual and their family. Wearing a brace, especially a full-time brace, is not a simple task.

a) Mental and social effects

Wearing a brace can have negative effects on the quality of life of individuals with AIS and is correlated with emotional stress, social isolation, poor body image, depression, and diminished exercise capacity.[49] These mental and social effects are not surprising since full-time wear requires the individual to wear their brace to school and social activities. Adolescents, especially, can find adherence to full-time brace wear to be challenging[50] because of the increased social awareness that accompany these years, such as not wanting to feel different from their peers and not wanting peers to know about their brace.

b) Physical discomfort

Most braces are rigid, and wearing one can be physically uncomfortable, causing an individual to feel hot or feel pressure on their torso. The brace may also limit their movement. These challenges can interfere with the individual's ability or desire to adhere to the prescribed brace wear time.

---

* Risk calculators are online assessment tools where an individual's specific information can be entered and the output shows the risk of treatment failure, based on research. Some calculators include brace wear time and show the risk of treatment failure in relation to the hours per day that a brace is worn.

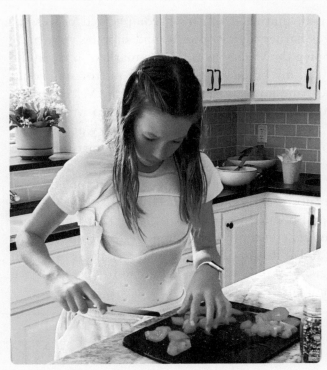

Lila wearing her brace during summer 2021.

Lila

Even with all the adjustments made to the brace, it felt big and very uncomfortable. I didn't want to wear it because it made me feel weird. I felt like I was wearing a big plastic shirt with some cushions in places where my spine had curved.

One of my least favorite parts about wearing a brace is how hot it is. You have to wear a shirt underneath it so the plastic doesn't irritate your skin. Even wearing an athletic-style shirt, as thin as possible, I just had to get used to the heat. I had to get a lot of other new clothes to accommodate the brace, too. When I first tried it on, my mom and I quickly realized that most shirts I owned would not work with it. We did a lot of shopping after that appointment and bought mostly baggy T-shirts and sweatshirts in darker colors. Unfortunately, tank tops didn't work because the brace rubbed into my armpits and quite a bit of the brace would show.

At first, I struggled with putting it on. It's a complicated process of opening it up (which is harder than it sounds) and slipping your body through it, then strapping the Velcro on at the pre-marked spots. In the beginning, I liked to put my brace on in front of a mirror so I could see my back and hands, and how far I needed to pull the Velcro straps. After a month or two, the brace became easier for me to wear and to put on and take off. The Velcro became a little less sticky and made a little less noise. It also became easier to put on without a mirror because the Velcro started leaving dents in the places where it needed to be fastened. One thing I really liked about the brace is that it forced me to sit up and work on my posture. I couldn't slouch because of the way the padding was placed and because it was plastic. Now that I no longer wear a brace, my mom is constantly reminding me to sit up straight. I'm a very active kid, and at the time I first got my brace I was in soccer, track, golf, swimming, and skiing, which meant I had to take my brace off quite often, especially in the summer.

Tana

Lila was instructed to wear the brace the majority of her waking hours. Both the doctor and orthotist recommended that she gradually work her way up to that over a week or two.

Her skin would become irritated from the brace rubbing, despite the shirts she wore underneath. I spent hours researching seamless shirt options to wear under the brace, and I bought probably 10 options of tees and tanks for her to try—in beige, white, and black. We had always hoped to find a tank top that would work with the brace, but her skin around her underarms would usually become irritated and she would have to switch to a T-shirt.

Lila worked hard at wearing her brace every waking moment that she could, but because she is a very active and athletic kid, we soon realized there were going to be times she simply could not wear it: swimming in the pool, at soccer practice, or skiing. Lila was happiest when moving, and we appreciated that her doctor told us to let her live her life, even with the brace. So Lila's philosophy on her daytime brace became that she would wear it every minute that she wasn't doing an activity that required her to remove it. Some days she would wear it for the full time, while other days were full of activities that meant she wore it less.

Even though Lila did not like the brace and thought it was hot and uncomfortable, she understood the importance of wearing it. But she really looked forward to the 24-hour brace break she was told to take before every doctor appointment—that was a highlight every few months!

Brace wear time adherence strategies

Strategies for improving brace wear time include:

- **Monitoring wear time and clinical counseling:** Technological advancements have allowed for the use of small commercial monitoring devices (e.g., a thermochron, a temperature logging sensor) to be embedded into spine braces to measure wear time.[51] The ability to accurately measure wear time has improved the ability to perform high-quality research that correlates wear time to outcome. [32,33,34,35] In addition, when brace wear time is monitored and the data is shown to individuals, families, and spine specialists, adherence improves.[52]
- **Co-designing the brace:** Having a visually pleasing brace (see Table 3.3.1) and involving the individual in the design process can increase wear time adherence and ease psychological challenges.[53]
- **Providing mental health support:** Adolescents and parents often seek online support to discuss their scoliosis and brace treatment.[54] Support groups and therapy or counseling may benefit individuals experiencing challenges with brace treatment.
- **Adhering to nighttime wear:** Prescribed nighttime wear eliminates many of the social challenges of full-time wear. For individuals with AIS, adherence to nighttime wear with a hypercorrective TLSO is higher than reports of full-time brace adherence.[55] It is important to note, however, that nighttime bracing may not be suitable for all individuals with idiopathic scoliosis.
- **Using flexible materials:** A brace made of flexible materials (also referred to as a soft brace) instead of rigid plastic can provide enhanced movement, lessen physical restrictions, and be more easily hidden underneath clothing.[49] How well flexible versus rigid braces

work in the treatment of scoliosis remains controversial, however, and requires further research,[49] and some medical centers may not prescribe them for curves that have shown to be progressive. As 3D printing technology advances and new materials emerge, it may be possible to use a more flexible brace that may improve comfort and allow more mobility while still providing the necessary amount of control to achieve bracing goals.

The spine specialist and orthotist will work with the individual and their family to establish the best brace option that matches their needs and goals. Additional resources are included in **Useful web resources**.

Lila

There is a lot I would tell someone with a back brace or the parent of a child with a brace. I suggest telling your teachers about your back brace so they can support any accommodations you may need. For me, I took my brace off during gym class because wearing it limited the activities I could participate in. To make sure I made it to the next class on time, I had to leave gym a few minutes early to have time to put the brace back on. Telling my teachers was also a good idea in case I was having a lot of back pain on a specific day and needed to visit the nurse or send a text message to my mom for any reason.

There are other small things I learned as well—things like bending down being quite tricky, especially to tie your shoes. Make sure that you put your brace on after tying your shoes, not before, and make sure you tie them well enough that they will stay tied.

Something kind of silly I did was to name my braces. Naming them made me feel a little happier and more positive about wearing a brace. I named the daytime one "Betsy, the big brown brace." The nighttime one I was later prescribed, which had a beautiful purple butterfly print, was "Petunia, the pretty purple brace." I didn't tell many of my friends I wore a brace, so if I had to talk to my parents about my brace while a friend or someone else was around, I would just refer to Betsy or Petunia.

Learning how to use the toilet also takes some getting used to. I was eventually able to do it without taking the brace off in the daytime, but with the nighttime brace I was not able to. It's important to always go right before bedtime so hopefully a middle-of-the-night trip isn't needed.

Tana

Most of Lila's school outfits were leggings with a dark-colored T-shirt and a hooded sweatshirt. Depending on the pants or leggings, she usually left the brace untucked and wore a longer shirt that covered its length. Warm days in summer were trickier to keep the brace concealed, but thankfully in Minnesota, there are not a lot of warm days when school is in session.

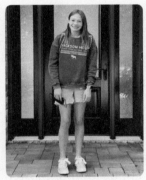

Lila on the first day of eighth grade, wearing her brace underneath a sweatshirt.

About six months after Lila received her daytime brace, we returned for a checkup with the doctor. That's when we learned that even though Lila was wearing her brace as much as she could, the curvature of her spine was continuing to worsen. The doctor suggested that Lila be fitted for a nighttime brace to be more aggressive in applying pressure to her spinal curves. This was a real disappointment for Lila. From that point, she wore her daytime brace during the day and slept in her nighttime brace. We met with the doctor two or three times a year to track Lila's growth and any changes in her curves. We also met with the orthotist at least as often, and sometimes every month or two. As Lila grew, and the rate of her growth began to pick up, she needed more frequent brace adjustments.

Casting

That which we persist in doing becomes easier—not that the nature of
the task has changed, but our ability to do has increased.

Ralph Waldo Emerson

Casting is typically only carried out for individuals with infantile idiopathic scoliosis (IIS). Cast treatment involves the application of plaster
to the torso. This plaster hardens into a cast, which applies corrective
forces and pressure to the spine to help improve the scoliosis curve and
to "guide" the spine to grow in a straight fashion. If complete correction is not possible, casting may also be used to prevent scoliosis curve
progression and delay surgery.

As shown in Figure 3.4.1, there is typically a cutout in the stomach area
and side or back of the cast to enhance comfort and curve correction.
Cutouts in the cast are placed on the opposite side of the scoliosis curve.
As the cast pushes on the spine to straighten it, the cutouts provide a
"relief" space for the body to shift into and the curve to straighten. The
cast may begin under the armpits, or it may extend over the shoulders.

Each cast is molded to the child's body, typically while the child is under general anesthesia. A special table is used to gently straighten the spine, then a spine specialist and casting specialist apply the plaster to the child's body and manually apply forces to derotate the spine while the plaster hardens, allowing the cast to form while the spine is in the corrected position. Once it is applied, the cast is not removed until it is time to apply the next cast or treatment ends. The cast is worn 24 hours a day for several months before it is removed and a new cast is applied. A cast is made of different materials than a brace, and it cannot be removed at home. Depending on age, a single cast may be worn for two to four months before it is replaced.[56]

This method of casting is referred to as Mehta casting. You may also hear it referred to as serial casting, elongation derotation flexion (EDF) casting, or derotational casting.

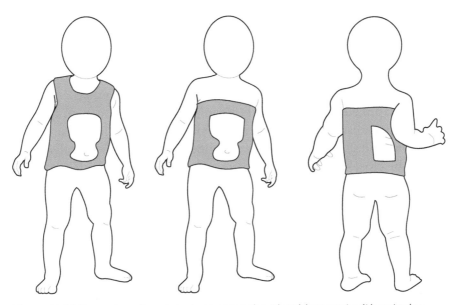

Figure 3.4.1 Examples of cast designs: over-the-shoulders cast with anterior opening (left), underarm cast with anterior opening (middle), underarm cast with posterior opening (right). Adapted with permission from Wolters Kluwer Health, Inc.: Sanders JO, D'Astous J, Fitzgerald M, et al. Derotational casting for progressive infantile scoliosis. *J Pediatr Orthop*, 29, 581-7, https://pubmed.ncbi.nlm.nih.gov/19700987/

When possible, delaying casting until after 12 months of age is recommended[57] to limit exposure to general anesthesia. The specific criteria for casting vary depending on the treatment center; here is one set of criteria for individuals with idiopathic scoliosis:*

- Age one to three years
- Cobb angle greater than 20 degrees
- RVAD greater than 20 degrees or rib phase 2

In contrast to bracing, which aims to prevent scoliosis curve progression, the goal of casting in children with idiopathic scoliosis under the age of two is to "cure" the condition (end treatment with a curve less than 10 degrees).[14] In children older than two years, there is a lower chance of scoliosis cure,[56] and a more realistic treatment goal may be to delay the need for surgery until the spine has achieved sufficient growth to allow good respiratory function in adulthood.[58]

Casting technique

Casting (application, removal, and reapplication) is often performed in an operating room while the child is under general anesthesia,† which may allow the child to be more relaxed and make manual correction easier and applied more effectively. If it is the child's first casting visit, the spine specialist may recommend a sedated MRI‡ to look for neural axis abnormalities. The child may stay one night at the hospital so that they can be closely monitored for any adverse reactions to the anesthesia or initial cast application, and to allow time to educate the family in cast care. For subsequent casting visits, the child generally goes home on the same day as the procedure.

A new cast will be applied regularly to accommodate growth. Typically, the cast removal and application of the new cast will be done on the same day. The timeline for casting change may vary among medical centers.

---

* Current criteria at Gillette Children's.

† Some treatment centers may perform casting while the child is awake. The method used typically depends on the spine specialist's preference and/or shared decision-making with the family.

‡ Young children often have difficulty staying still for an MRI. An MRI done while the child is sedated may be the best option. Performing this MRI on the same day as a casting procedure reduces the number of anesthesia exposures.

A typical timeline is:[59]

- Under three years old—casting change every two months
- Three years old—casting change every three months

Duration of casting treatment

Many families wonder how long their casting experience will last. This varies based on the child and the status of their scoliosis curve (i.e., their progression or improvement during treatment). Resolution of the scoliosis curve typically takes one year or more of serial casting.[*58]

Ending casting treatment

Casting may end for the following reasons:

- The curve improves to a Cobb angle less than 15 degrees as measured on two consecutive standing X-rays, after the child has been out of their cast for a few hours.
- The casting is not tolerated (e.g., skin breakdown).
- The family desires to discontinue casting treatment.
- The Cobb angle progresses to greater than 50 degrees; at this curve size, surgery may be recommended.

After serial casting, the child may transition immediately to wearing a brace (see section 3.3). This decision will be made based on the child's current curve size and their anticipated risk of further progression after treatment. The child will need to be followed closely after ending casting treatment, with regular visits every four to six months to monitor the curvature for signs of progression. Children who have a Cobb angle greater than 10 degrees at the end of casting are at a significantly higher risk of needing future treatment for their scoliosis than those who have a Cobb angle less than 10 degrees.[60]

---

* This research included individuals with idiopathic scoliosis, syndromic scoliosis, and scoliosis secondary to neural axis abnormalities.

Cast efficacy

Measurements for treatment success are not well defined, but the following criteria have been used:

- Having an out-of-cast Cobb angle less than 15 degrees on an upright (standing or sitting) X-ray at the most recent follow-up.[61,62]
- Delaying the need for scoliosis surgery until adolescence (age 10 to 19 years old)—may be considered a "good" outcome.[60]
- Avoiding the need for any future scoliosis surgery—may be considered an "excellent" outcome.[60]

Casting has been shown to be safe and effective.[63,64,65] Some factors that are frequently associated with casting success include:

- **Age at initial casting:** Casting success has been highest in individuals with idiopathic scoliosis who undergo their initial casting prior to 18 months of age.[61] Thus, early diagnosis of scoliosis and early initiation of casting treatment are important.[56,58,59,62]
- **Pretreatment Cobb angle:** Casting success is highest in individuals with a smaller initial Cobb angle.[58,59,62] Although the exact Cobb angle is not widely agreed upon, Sanders and colleagues have reported that curves of less than 50 to 60 degrees have better casting outcomes than curves greater than 60 degrees.[58]
- **Initial cast correction:** Greater correction of the curve (i.e., smaller curve size) in the first cast is associated with an increased success rate.[62]

Up to 49 percent of individuals with IIS have a Cobb angle of 15 degrees or less after casting, with up to 71 percent experiencing significant curve correction.[57] The average amount of Cobb angle correction is 25 degrees.[63]

Casting challenges

In contrast to a brace, a cast does not need to be put on and taken off daily. This ensures better treatment adherence, and many families may prefer casting treatment as it lessens the burden of enforcing brace wear on a young child. However, casting treatment can also be challenging for children and their families.

a) Risk of complications

As with any treatment, casting comes with the risk of complications. The most common complications include skin irritation and temporary respiratory (breathing) difficulties.[63]

- Pressure wounds may develop during casting, especially in children who have a limited ability to communicate their discomfort.[57] Because of this risk, it is important that the cast be well padded.[57]
- While casts have cutouts to assist with breathing, it is possible that children may find it difficult to breathe deeply or cough, especially in times of respiratory illness.

It is important for parents to closely monitor their child for signs of skin irritation (in areas of the body that are visible, such as the armpits) or respiratory challenges during cast treatment. The child's skin will also be closely examined during cast removal and new cast application.

b) Effects on health-related quality of life

Cast treatment may negatively impact the child's or the parent's health-related quality of life (HRQOL).* Specifically, casting is associated with psychosocial stress,[66] which may or may not improve after ending cast treatment.[66,67]

Casting presents other challenges that can disrupt normal family activities. For instance, most casts cannot get wet (an exception is a waterproof cast that some medical centers may use). This limitation poses challenges for hygiene and prevents children from participating in activities such as bathing or swimming. Other activities may also be limited; for example, it is ill advised for a child wearing a cast to jump on a trampoline with other children as it may harm others if a collision were to occur.

---

* An individual's or a group's perceived physical and mental health over time.[68]

c) Repeat anesthesia exposure

Cast removal and reapplication are often performed under general anesthesia. Repeated exposure to general anesthesia has raised questions regarding potential negative impact during early development. In 2016, the US Food and Drug Administration (FDA) issued a warning that general anesthesia in children younger than three years of age may affect brain development.[69] This warning was based on research in animal subjects, not humans, and has not been clearly supported by quality research in children.[69]

While this is an area of active research and not yet conclusive, it does demonstrate that multiple general anesthesia exposures in early childhood may be accompanied by an increased, moderate risk of negative impact on neurodevelopment (impact on brain development that leads to cognitive and/or behavioral deficits).[70] There is much unknown in this area, including the relationship of frequency and duration of anesthesia use with these potential risks.[70] Limiting the duration, dose, and frequency of general anesthesia exposure in early childhood is recommended, given the uncertainty of long-term developmental effects.[70]

Spine specialists recommend pursuing casting only when they believe the benefits outweigh the potential risks of general anesthesia exposure. Some medical centers may advocate for performing casting procedures while the child is awake to avoid the use of general anesthesia,[71] but this can be difficult for young children.

Cast holidays

Some medical centers may allow "cast holidays," during which the child wears a TLSO instead of a cast or takes a break from treatment altogether. This commonly occurs during the summer months[72] and is done in an effort to improve quality of life. During a cast holiday, the child can move more freely and participate in activities such as swimming and bathing. While there may be a psychosocial benefit to a cast holiday, research shows that children with early-onset scoliosis (EOS) who take a cast holiday within the first 18 months of treatment are less likely to achieve correction of their scoliosis, to less than 15 degrees, compared with children who do not.[72]

At Gillette Children's, spine specialists do not typically recommend traditional cast holidays. For some children, they may allow a week break from the cast. However, it has not been studied if this week-long break has an impact on treatment outcomes.

Physical therapy

We are what we repeatedly do.
Excellence, then, is not an act, but a habit.
Aristotle

"Physical therapists provide services that develop, maintain, and restore a person's maximum movement and functional ability."[73] This is done through treatment methods including therapeutic exercise, massage, assistive devices, and patient education. Physical therapists have different titles in different countries: in many countries they are called physiotherapists. In this book, the terms "physical therapist" and "physical therapy" are used.

There are two types of physical therapy (or physiotherapy) commonly used for individuals with scoliosis:

- **Traditional physical therapy:** Therapy available to all individuals.
- **Physical therapy scoliosis-specific exercises (PSSE):** A type of physical therapy available to individuals with scoliosis that aims to help the individual control their posture through stretching, strengthening, posture corrections, breathing exercises, and education. It is

recommended that individuals be at least 10 years old to participate in PSSE.

The type of physical therapy recommended will depend on the individual's and family's goals. Therapy may occur before, during, or after other scoliosis treatment and is considered an add-on or complement to other treatment (observation, bracing, casting, surgery). In other words, physical therapy may be a helpful addition to the current scoliosis treatment plan but should not replace it.

Traditional physical therapy

Traditional physical therapy for individuals with scoliosis may be appropriate to address back pain, postural concerns, or strength imbalances, though the goal is not to treat scoliosis specifically and thus has not been shown to improve scoliosis curves.[74]

Physical therapy often requires a referral by a medical professional, such as a primary care provider or spine specialist. During the initial evaluation, the physical therapist will work with the individual and their family to form therapy goals and create care plans to help the individual achieve these goals.

Physical therapy scoliosis-specific exercises

Physical therapy scoliosis-specific exercises (PSSE) is a type of physical therapy that aims to help the individual with scoliosis control their posture. It consists of the following:[75]

- Self-correction of posture in three dimensions
- Training in activities of daily living*
- Stabilization of the corrected posture
- Patient education

---

* Activities of daily living are essential daily tasks that most young and healthy individuals can perform without help.[76]

PSSE is performed with a physical therapist who has been specially trained in physical therapy for scoliosis. While the methods of PSSE have been used in treatment since the early 1920s,[77] there is limited research showing their effects on preventing progression, whether in isolation or in combination with a brace. As such, there is a lack of agreement among spine specialists on ideal candidates, dosing prescriptions, and short- or long-term outcomes.

The following criteria may be used as a general guideline to identify appropriate PSSE candidates; different treatment centers may have different criteria:

- Nonsurgical individuals who:
  o Are older than 10 years
  o Have a Cobb angle of 15 degrees or greater
  o Have back pain not associated with injury or trauma
- Post-surgery individuals who need additional support in their recovery and who have:
  o Postural imbalance
  o Lumbar curve that has not been operated on (surgery was performed on other regions of the spine, not the lumbar region)
  o Difficulty with pain management

Starting PSSE

When a spine specialist thinks an individual would benefit from PSSE, they will make a referral to a physical therapist with specialized training for an initial PSSE evaluation. During this initial evaluation, the physical therapist will review the individual's medical history and X-rays, and perform an evaluation of their range of motion (ROM),* posture, strength, functional mobility, respiratory function, and pain.[78] The physical therapist will create a customized plan based on this information. The number of sessions per week, length of the sessions, and overall time spent in PSSE treatment will vary depending on the treatment center.

---

* The ROM is a measure of joint flexibility. The actual ROM through which a joint can be passively moved is measured in degrees. An instrument called a goniometer is used to measure the ROM of a joint.

A typical plan might be PSSE sessions of 60 minutes each scheduled one or two times per week for three or four months.

During PSSE, the physical therapist helps the individual identify their optimal posture given the shape of the scoliosis curve. The individual can then focus on stabilizing the muscles around the spine to keep that optimal posture and integrate the posture into daily activities. Images from a PSSE session can be seen in Figure 3.5.1.

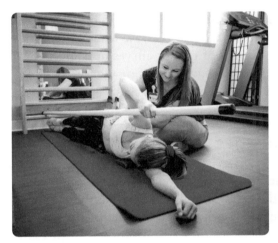 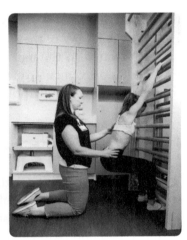

Figure 3.5.1 Exercises during a PSSE session.

PSSE home program

The individual will also be assigned an individualized exercise plan to follow at home between the scheduled PSSE sessions. Once an individual reaches skeletal maturity, they are instructed to continue with a maintenance home exercise program through adolescence and adulthood to promote spine health and mobility.

Families can purchase specialized equipment to assist with their at-home PSSE program if they have the space. This equipment ranges in cost.

PSSE efficacy

There is still a lack of high-quality research supporting the effectiveness of PSSE in the treatment of AIS (and a general lack of research addressing the application of PSSE in other age groups), but studies of individuals with AIS show that PSSE helps to stabilize the scoliosis curve (slow or stop curve progression)—at least in the first few years of treatment—and improve quality of life, functional activity, muscle strength and general conditioning, mental health, body image, and satisfaction with care.[79,80,81] There is no consensus on its effect on pain.[79,81,82] However, with any of these studies, it is hard to know whether the findings are related to the natural history of milder curves and short-term postural improvements during X-ray examination or whether there is truly long-term stabilization or improvement of curves.

Physical therapy challenges

When discussing physical therapy with a spine specialist, challenges such as access and time should be considered. Traditional physical therapy is more widely accessible for families, in contrast to PSSE which requires specially trained physical therapists. Additionally, physical therapy is time-intensive, and successful treatment requires attending many sessions as well as performing assigned exercises at home.

Alternative and complementary treatments

We keep moving forward, opening new doors, and doing new things, because we're curious and curiosity keeps leading us down new paths.

Walt Disney

Alternative and complementary treatments are treatments that are not part of conventional health care. Alternative treatments may be used in place of conventional medicine, while complementary treatments are used together with conventional medicine.[83]

Families may consider alternative and complementary treatments for several reasons, including:

- Hearing about a treatment option in the media or from family and friends
- Wanting to try all treatment options available
- Wanting to complement or increase the effectiveness of present treatment
- Wanting to relieve symptoms (such as pain)

If the parent-professional relationship is good, parents should be able to discuss these options with the medical professionals who treat their child. Both parents and professionals should be guided by the best research evidence available. Spine specialists may recommend or approve some of these treatment options as complementary to other scoliosis treatment (observation, bracing, casting, surgery) as a helpful add-on to the current scoliosis treatment plan, but they should not replace the current treatment plan.

Table 3.6.1 lists common alternative and complementary treatments.

Table 3.6.1 Alternative and complementary treatments

TREATMENT	DESCRIPTION OF TREATMENT	EVIDENCE SUPPORTING TREATMENT IN SCOLIOSIS
Chiropractic therapy	A type of therapy involving the diagnosis, treatment, and prevention of conditions involving the musculoskeletal system. Chiropractic therapy focuses on manual treatments such as spinal adjustment and joint or soft-tissue manipulation.	There is a lack of evidence that chiropractic therapy can be used to treat scoliosis, and current research suggests spinal manipulation does not influence progression of the scoliosis curve.[84] Additionally, medical professionals have expressed concerns about the safety of chiropractic therapy in scoliosis; research has found that mild side effects such as muscle soreness, neck pain, back pain, and headaches are common after treatment.*[85]
Yoga	A practice that includes specific body postures, breath control, and meditation.	Yoga may help to strengthen muscles and alleviate problems such as back pain; however, there is no research to support the effectiveness of yoga in treating scoliosis.
Pilates	A type of exercise designed to improve physical strength, flexibility, posture, and mental awareness.	Pilates may help to strengthen muscles, but there is no research to support the effectiveness of Pilates in treating scoliosis.

* It is highly recommended that individuals who pursue chiropractic care also continue to see their spine specialist regularly for objective measures of their scoliosis outcomes.

Cont'd.

TREATMENT	DESCRIPTION OF TREATMENT	EVIDENCE SUPPORTING TREATMENT IN SCOLIOSIS
Acupuncture	A treatment that involves inserting thin needles into the skin at specific points.	Acupuncture is a safe treatment and may have some effect when performed with other conventional scoliosis treatments,[86] but further research is needed.
Massage	A therapy that involves applying pressure to muscles, generally using the hands, to relieve pain and tension.	Massage may be helpful for individuals with scoliosis who have back pain. However, there is no research that indicates massage may have any effect on the scoliosis curve. Following scoliosis surgery, massage is safe and may help relieve muscle discomfort. It is important for the massage professional to be made aware of any surgical implants present in the spine.

Alternative and complementary treatments for scoliosis have varying levels of scientific evidence to support their use. Just as spine specialists and families weigh the potential benefits and risks of traditional treatment options based on the level of scientific evidence available, so too must they weigh the potential benefits and risks with alternative and complementary treatments.

Key points Chapter 3

- Nonsurgical treatment of scoliosis is treatment that does not require surgery.
- The overall goal of nonsurgical treatment is to slow or stop curve progression to prevent or delay surgery.
- Observation for scoliosis requires regular X-rays and clinical exams with a spine specialist.
- Candidates for observation are deemed to have a low risk of scoliosis curve progression.
- The most common type of spinal brace is the thoraco-lumbo-sacral orthosis (TLSO). It is typically made from molded, rigid plastic that extends from the armpits down past the hips.
- The two types of TLSOs are full-time (prescribed for 18 to 23 hours per day) and nighttime hypercorrective (prescribed for 8 to 12 hours per day).
- In most cases of idiopathic scoliosis, wearing a brace does not improve or straighten the curve. Instead, the goal of treatment is to prevent the curve from progressing.
- Successful bracing treatment in AIS is correlated with wear time.
- Cast treatment involves the application of plaster to the torso, molded to the child's body. This plaster hardens into a cast.
- Casting is typically carried out only for individuals with IIS.
- The goal of casting in children with idiopathic scoliosis under the age of two years is to "cure" scoliosis (end treatment with a curve less than 10 degrees).
- Physical therapy scoliosis-specific exercises (PSSE) is a type of physical therapy that aims to help the individual with scoliosis control their posture.
- Physical therapy may occur before, during, or after other scoliosis treatment and is considered an add-on or complement to other scoliosis treatment.
- Alternative and complementary treatments (chiropractic therapy, yoga, Pilates, acupuncture, massage) may be helpful add-ons to the current scoliosis treatment plan but should not replace the current treatment plan.

Chapter 4

Scoliosis surgery

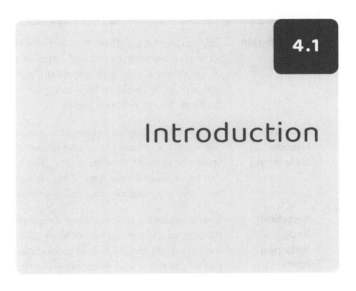

4.1

Introduction

*You see things and say "Why?"; but I dream things
that never were and I say "Why not?"*
George Bernard Shaw

Surgical treatment of scoliosis is also referred to as operative treatment, or scoliosis surgery. "Scoliosis surgery" is the term used in this book. The types of scoliosis surgery addressed in this chapter include:

- Spinal fusion
- Growth-friendly treatment
- Vertebral body tethering (VBT)

See Table 4.1.1.

Table 4.1.1 Description of scoliosis surgeries

TREATMENT	DESCRIPTION OF SURGERY
Spinal fusion	Fusing (joining together) two or more vertebrae in the spine to stop curve progression and improve the angle of the curve (decrease the Cobb angle), typically performed using metal rods and screws or hooks to hold the spine in a corrected position and facilitate fusion between bones.
Growth-friendly treatment	Improving the angle of the scoliosis curve (decreasing the Cobb angle) by using metal rods and screws or hooks to stabilize the spine above and below the curve. The length of the metal rods can be expanded over time. This includes traditional growing rods and magnetically controlled growing rods (MCGRs).
Vertebral body tethering (VBT)	Inserting screws and attaching a rope (tether), which is under tension, to the convex side of the scoliosis curve (the outside of the curve). As the individual grows, the growth on the convex side of the curve is slowed, allowing the concave side (the inside of the curve) to continue to grow and allowing the spine to straighten.

The specific goals of each scoliosis surgery differ, but the overall goals of scoliosis surgery are to:

- Stop curve progression
- Improve the spinal curve (decrease the Cobb angle)
- Achieve a balanced spine and posture

This chapter also discusses halo gravity traction, which is a multistage treatment for severe scoliosis to stretch and straighten the spine and soft tissues (skin, muscle, ligaments) *prior* to scoliosis surgery (see section 4.7).

Scoliosis surgeries are overwhelmingly safe, and spine specialists recommend a surgery only if they believe the benefits outweigh the potential risks for the individual. But there are risks with any surgery. Surgical risks are things that may go wrong while in or shortly after surgery while the individual is still in the hospital (in-hospital complications). Long-term complications are problems that may occur after the individual has been discharged from the hospital and may develop over the course of months or even years following surgery. Risk management is the highest priority for hospitals and spine specialists, and many safety measures are in place to maximize safety. However, it is important for families to be aware of these risks and discuss them as part of the shared decision-making process.

Tana

The discussion of Lila potentially needing surgery occurred about 18 months after she had begun bracing. Nothing was different with Lila's spine as far as she was concerned—she didn't have pain, and the only discomfort was generally caused by the brace. Her curvature was noticeable only when she wore a swimsuit, but family members commented that they would never have known that she had scoliosis if they hadn't been told. But at this appointment, the doctor shared his concern that Lila's spinal curves had continued to worsen. She was also 13 years old and had not yet had her large growth spurt. That meant her curves were likely to continue to worsen and she would likely need surgery at some point.

Getting that news at this appointment derailed all plans we had for the day. Even though it was an early-morning appointment, Lila did not make it to school that day, and I didn't make it to work. She had an additional test or two as ordered by the doctor, more meetings with the doctor, and another with the orthotist for brace adjustments.

Lila

Talk of surgery first came up at one of my appointments when the doctor said that the brace might not be doing enough for my back and that the curve degrees were still increasing. At a later appointment, the doctor told me about the different types of surgeries I could get, one being a tether (VBT), which is basically a small rope inside of your back adjusting the curve over time. The other option is the fusion, which is having a metal rod placed in your back, which sounded very scary in my opinion (even though it is known to be effective and safe). The doctor said I was the perfect candidate for the tether surgery since I had the right amount of growth left.

On the way home from that appointment, my mom asked me how I felt about getting surgery. I was emotional because I felt bad for everyone having to do so much to help me, but I answered, "Good, because everyone is doing everything that they can to help me." My parents, still to this day, like to tell me how brave and strong I am for being so positive even though I have had to deal with a lot of things that other kids will never have to. I have always thought that I was given all the special things because I can handle it. Now looking back on it, I am so glad that I was given all these obstacles to deal with because I learned that life isn't perfect. I also learned how to deal with that, to stay positive, and to understand that all these experiences will make me a better person. I want to help others when I am older because I want to give back to all the people who have helped me.

USEFUL WEB RESOURCES

Preparing for surgery

It's a terrible thing, I think, in life to wait until you're ready. I have this feeling now that actually no one is ever ready to do anything. There is almost no such thing as ready. There is only now. And you may as well do it now. Generally speaking, now is as good a time as any.

Hugh Laurie

Preparing for surgery can be overwhelming. The following list describes appointments, procedures, and advice that may help prepare:

- **Initial discussions:** Initial discussions about surgery can begin at clinical visits weeks or months in advance. Take notes at appointments (using a notebook or a notes app) and ask for information in writing where possible. This information can then be referred to later.
- **Presurgical appointments:** It is standard to have presurgical appointments with a spine specialist and primary care provider. The goals of these appointments are to ensure the individual is healthy, is prepared for surgery, and knows what to expect.
- **Questions to ask:** Many families find it helpful to keep a list of questions that come up in the days before surgery. Bring notes to the

preoperative appointments and/or surgery. It can also be helpful to keep notes during the hospital stay to keep track of things that are happening and write down additional questions that may come up.

- **Presurgical imaging:** Prior to surgery, the spine specialist may order imaging specific to the surgery type. Advanced imaging such as CT scans, MRI scans, or additional spine X-rays may be ordered.
- **Pulmonary (lung) function testing:** Scoliosis can impact the function of the lungs (see section 2.4), so lung function may be measured before and at least six months after surgery to assess lung capacity and effectiveness. A pulmonary function test is a simple, noninvasive procedure that involves the individual breathing into a tube connected to a device called a spirometer.
- **Hospital tours:** Most hospitals, especially children's hospitals, will have an option to take a tour of the facility before surgery. This can help lessen stress for both the child and their family. It will also give families a chance to ask additional questions about the hospital stay, such as who can visit and when, what comfort items may be brought in (stuffed animals, special blankets, etc.), what food is available, and any other room-related questions the family may have. If an in-person tour is not an option, ask about virtual or video tours, which many hospitals offer.
- **Child life specialists:** Child life specialists are pediatric health care professionals who work with children and adolescents and their families to help them cope with the challenges of hospitalization, illness, and disability. Child life specialists can work in age-appropriate ways to prepare the child for surgery. They can also assist with strategies to help siblings and prepare them for what their brother or sister will look like after surgery, particularly if they will be visiting the hospital. This role may have a different title in other countries.
- **Counseling:** The child may be referred for psychological counseling because surgery can be a significant source of anxiety for individuals and families. Seeking counseling in preparation for surgery may help alleviate some of this anxiety and identify coping strategies.
- **Cleaning the body before surgery:** The child may be asked to wash their hair and body with special antibacterial soap the day before or the day of surgery. This helps to prevent infection.
- **Eating and drinking before surgery:** Families will be given specific instructions on when the child must stop eating and drinking before surgery. It is important to follow these exactly. For young children,

it may be helpful to check the car seat and back seat area for stray food or bottles before leaving for the hospital, especially if the child is at an age where they may grab items and put them in their mouth independently.

The patient and their family will be instructed to arrive at a specific time on the day of surgery (e.g., one and a half hours prior to surgery). After arrival and check-in, the patient and family will be taken to a presurgical area where nurses will measure the patient's vitals, including heart rate, oxygen level, blood pressure, and temperature. Members of the patient's care team will discuss the surgery and make sure the patient and family feel comfortable and prepared. Then, once in the operating room, general anesthesia will be administered to the patient so they fall asleep prior to the start of surgery. A urinary catheter will be inserted once the patient is asleep in the operating room and prior to the start of surgery. This small tube drains urine from the bladder during and after surgery.

For more information about preparing for surgery, see **Useful web resources.**

Spinal fusion

It always seems impossible until it's done.

Nelson Mandela

Spinal fusion is the most common type of scoliosis surgery; it has been performed for the longest period of all surgeries and has the most studies assessing outcomes. It involves fusing (joining together) two or more vertebrae in the spine, typically all the bones in the curvature. For single curves, typically 7 or 8 vertebrae are fused, and for double curves, typically 10 to 12 vertebrae are fused.

Typically, metal rods and screws (termed "instrumentation" or "implants") are used to straighten the spine, hold it in the straighter position, and facilitate fusion between the bones (see Figure 4.3.1).

The process of fusing vertebrae eliminates movement between them and enhances stability of the spine, keeping it straight. Spinal fusion halts growth of the spine in the fused areas. The rods and screws are typically not removed from the body unless there are complications.

Spinal fusion can be performed using an anterior approach, posterior approach, or a combination of both. With an anterior approach, the surgeon accesses the spine through the front or side of the body. With a posterior approach, the surgeon accesses the spine through the back of the body. Posterior spinal fusion is by far the most common approach.

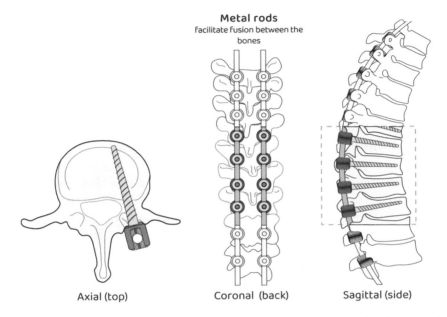

Metal rods
facilitate fusion between the bones

Axial (top)   Coronal (back)   Sagittal (side)

Figure 4.3.1 Posterior spinal fusion placement of screws and metal rods connected to the screws.

Spinal fusion goals

The primary goals of spinal fusion are to:

- Stop curve progression
- Improve the spinal curve (decrease the Cobb angle)
- Achieve a balanced spine and posture

The spine surgeon aims to provide a durable and long-lasting curve correction and minimize the likelihood of the individual requiring another spinal surgery in the future, while also attempting to fuse as few vertebrae as possible in order to preserve as much motion in the spine as possible.

From the individual's point of view, benefits of spinal fusion include cosmetic improvements due to enhanced symmetry of the torso and less rotation of the rib cage. Individuals are also taller after spinal fusion due to the straightening of the scoliosis curve.

Who is a candidate for spinal fusion?

Spinal fusion halts the growth of the spine and is generally not an appropriate surgery for very young children. The general recommendation is that spinal fusion should be delayed until children reach 10 years of age.[14] However, the ideal age for the individual will vary based on the point at which their lung development will enable them to enter adulthood without significant pulmonary compromise.

One factor used to assess readiness for spinal fusion is thoracic height (the length of the thoracic region of the spine); however, there is no agreed minimum thoracic height required for successful fusion.[14,87]

The ideal candidate for spinal fusion meets the following criteria:

- Is at least 10 years of age or has achieved a sufficient thoracic height[14]
- Has a Cobb angle equal to or greater than 50 degrees

These criteria may differ among medical centers.

Spinal fusion timing

Because idiopathic scoliosis is usually not symptomatic during adolescence (e.g., no back pain or shortness of breath), some individuals may choose to forgo recommended spinal fusion until they experience symptoms in adulthood. However, spine specialists often advocate for spinal fusion surgery in adolescence instead of adulthood. As discussed in section 2.4, spine specialists recommend surgery to help the individual avoid the long-term effects of untreated scoliosis (preventive) as opposed to operating to reverse existing symptoms.

Additionally, outcomes may be better when surgery is done during adolescence rather than young adulthood, including less blood loss, increased curve correction, and fewer vertebrae operated on.[88] Surgery and recovery for an adolescent may also be more convenient and practical than for an adult with competing responsibilities (time off from work, taking care of children, etc.). Finally, preventing, rather than reversing, the complications associated with large scoliosis curves, such as worsening pulmonary function or back pain, is typically safer and more successful. Once these complications have developed, it becomes much more difficult to reverse them.

What happens during a spinal fusion?

A spinal fusion is performed in an operating room while the patient is under general anesthesia. The duration of the surgery varies, but it may be anywhere from three to eight hours. Factors that affect duration include the number of vertebrae being fused, the size of the scoliosis curves, the size of the patient, and the surgical approach (posterior spinal fusion versus anterior spinal fusion or combined).

a) Selection of fusion levels

You may hear spine specialists talk about "fusion levels." This term refers to the spine region and the location (specific vertebra) within that region. For example, "L1" refers to the first vertebra in the lumbar region of the spine. The "upper instrumented vertebra" is the highest vertebra (closest to the head) that is instrumented (has screws or hooks), and the "lower instrumented vertebra" refers to the lowest vertebra (closest to the tailbone) that is instrumented. Most vertebrae between the upper and lower instrumented vertebrae may have implants (screws or hooks) in them, and metal rods connect all vertebrae from the upper to the lower instrumented vertebra.

The number of vertebrae that are fused varies depending on the scoliosis curve location, size, flexibility, and balance of the spine. This decision can be aided by specialized presurgical imaging including X-rays that demonstrate the amount of flexibility within the spine. The selection of fusion levels is planned to obtain optimal short-term and long-term outcomes.

Fusing vertebrae will reduce the range of motion through the fused area. Surgeons are thoughtful in selecting the fewest number of vertebrae to operate on to achieve a successful scoliosis curve improvement (decrease the Cobb angle) while maximizing the remaining range of motion and flexibility in the spine. This is an example of the many factors that spine specialists consider when deciding fusion levels.

b) Supporting fusion levels

To promote fusion of vertebrae, bone graft material is used. Bone graft is the addition of transplanted bone to an area to help repair and rebuild bone. In spinal fusion, the bone graft acts as a biologic scaffolding, promoting the growth of new bone between the vertebrae (joining the vertebrae together). Bone grafts can be obtained from the area of the surgery or another area in the individual's body, such as the pelvis or ribs (termed "autograft"), or they can come from a donor or synthetic source (termed "allograft"). Additionally, instrumentation helps to retain spinal alignment while the fusion forms.

Figure 4.3.2 shows X-ray images from before and after a posterior spinal fusion.

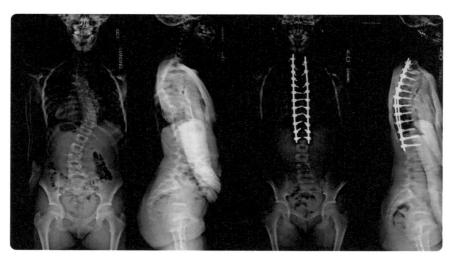

Figure 4.3.2 X-rays from before (left) and after (right) posterior spinal fusion. In this case, the fusion included 12 levels from T2 to L1 (second thoracic vertebra to first lumbar vertebra).

After a spinal fusion, the individual will stay in the hospital until they meet milestones required to discharge and go home (see section 4.6). The typical length of hospital stay varies depending on the individual's condition and needs. Typically, individuals with idiopathic scoliosis are discharged after one or two days.

Spinal fusion surgical risks and long-term complications

The surgical risks for spinal fusion include:

- **Neurologic injury:** There is a risk of neurologic injury (injury to the spinal cord or nerves resulting in temporary or permanent loss of function or sensation) during scoliosis surgery. During surgery, motor and sensory function* is carefully monitored in real time. This is referred to as "intraoperative neurophysiological monitoring" (IONM) or "intraoperative monitoring" (IOM). If any change in motor or sensory function is detected, the spine specialist immediately assesses the situation and takes appropriate action.
- **Postoperative infection:** There is a risk of infection after surgery, particularly infection of the surgical incision. To decrease this risk, patients are instructed to wash with an antibacterial soap prior to surgery, surgery is performed using sterile techniques, and the patient receives IV antibiotics immediately before, during, and after surgery.
- **Excessive blood loss:** To decrease the risk of excessive blood loss, patients are given medication during surgery. At some hospitals, blood that is lost during surgery may be collected in a "cell saver." This collected blood can be concentrated and returned to the patient if necessary. Also, when necessary, donor blood transfusions may be performed.
- **General anesthesia:** While general anesthesia is considered very safe, there are risks to its use. Most side effects are minor and temporary.[89] Risks include nausea, chills, vomiting, confusion, and a sore throat from the breathing tube used when a patient is under

---

* Motor function refers to the ability to move, while sensory function refers to the ability to receive and interpret information from the environment (e.g., vision, touch).

general anesthesia.[89] More information about general anesthesia risks is included in **Useful web resources.**

Data from a US nationwide database showed an in-hospital spinal fusion complication rate of 8 percent for individuals with adolescent idiopathic scoliosis (AIS).[90]

The following are potential long-term complications of spinal fusion:

- **Pseudoarthrosis:** The failure of fusion; that is, the failure of the bones to unite properly
- **Instrumentation-related complications:** Loosening of implanted instrumentation, migration of instrumentation (shifting from intended location), or any other malfunction of instrumentation
- **Proximal junctional kyphosis (PJK):** Hyperkyphosis that develops above the upper instrumented vertebra,*[91] which can weaken the connection between the screws and bone, causing the screws to pull out of the bone and/or for the instrumentation to be prominent (visible) through the skin
- **Development of additional spinal curvatures:** The development of additional curvature above and below the surgical instrumentation (metal rods and screws or hooks); also referred to as "adding on"

Data from an international multicenter register shows that long-term complications for individuals with AIS were reported by 10 percent of individuals a minimum of 10 years after spinal fusion.[92] Ideally, spinal fusion is the final (or for many, the only) surgery required to correct an individual's scoliosis. However, some long-term complications of spinal fusion may lead to additional surgery. This is called "reoperation." Studies of posterior spinal fusion in individuals with AIS reported a reoperation rate of 2 percent three or more years after surgery[93] and 8 percent at a minimum of 10 years after surgery.[92]

---

* The upper instrumented vertebra is the highest vertebra (closest to the head) that is instrumented (has screws or hooks).

Growth-friendly treatment

The past never returns, but the character of the future can be determined, in part, by what is done in the present.
Owen Harding Wangensteen

Growth-friendly treatment refers to surgical instrumentation (metal rods and screws or hooks) placed in the spine without fusing the vertebrae or with limited fusion. The instrumentation can be attached to the vertebrae, ribs, or pelvis and is implanted above and below the scoliosis curve. The length of the metal rods can be expanded over time to limit curve progression while allowing a child to continue to grow. These rods can be thought of as an "internal brace" to prevent curve progression. This section addresses two growth-friendly treatments: traditional growing rods and magnetically controlled growing rods (MCGRs). See Table 4.4.1.

Table 4.4.1 Growth-friendly treatments

TYPE	EXPLANATION	LENGTHENING PROCESS AFTER INITIAL SURGERY
Traditional growing rods	Metal rods are manually lengthened during surgical procedures under general anesthesia.	• Invasive (i.e., requires surgery) • Surgically lengthened every four to six months
Magnetically controlled growing rods (MCGRs)	Adjustable rods are lengthened via a magnetic remote control in clinic.	• Noninvasive (i.e., does not require surgery) • Lengthened in clinic every two to three months with a remote control

Growth-friendly treatment goals

Growth-friendly treatment provides scoliosis curve management while allowing the spine and chest to continue growing to an appropriate size to support adult-size heart and lungs. The primary goals of growth-friendly treatment are to:

- Prevent significant curve progression while allowing spine and chest wall growth
- Partially correct the spinal curve (decrease the Cobb angle)
- Maintain a balanced spine and posture

Who is a candidate for growth-friendly treatment?

The ideal candidate for growth-friendly treatment meets the following criteria:

- Younger than 10 years old and/or has insufficient thoracic height for spinal fusion
- Cobb angle of 50 degrees or greater

These criteria may differ among medical centers.

Traditional growing rods

Traditional growing rods are metal rods that are manually lengthened during surgery under general anesthesia. They are attached to the spine via screws or hooks. See Figure 4.4.1.

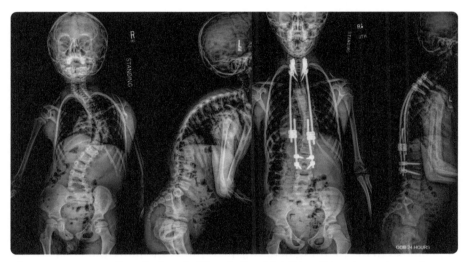

Figure 4.4.1 X-rays from before (left) and after (right) traditional growing rod surgery.

Traditional growing rods were the first type of growth-friendly surgery available, but because using them requires frequent surgeries for the lengthening, they have become less popular than MCGRs (see below). Currently, traditional growing rods are typically offered only to individuals who are not candidates for MCGRs. Reasons that traditional growing rods may be offered instead of MCGRs include:

- **Curve type:** Individuals with particularly stiff curves or hyperkyphosis are not ideal candidates for MCGRs (more force can be applied in traditional growing rod lengthening than MCGRs).
- **High body mass index (BMI):** Individuals with a high BMI have a greater distance between the placed rods and the surface of their skin, making it difficult to achieve the magnetic force required to lengthen the MCGRs with a remote control.
- **Patient size:** Traditional growing rods can be effectively placed in very small children, whereas the shortest MCGRs may be too long for them.

The initial traditional growing rod surgery is performed in an operating room while the patient is under general anesthesia. The duration of the surgery varies but may take two to five hours. During this initial surgery, screws or hooks are attached to the vertebrae or ribs above and below the curve. Two rods are attached to the screws, and the spine is moved into a straighter position.

After implantation of traditional growing rods, the length of hospital stay will vary. Individuals will recover in the hospital until they meet milestones required to discharge and go home (see section 4.6). A typical hospital stay is two days. Following the initial traditional growing rod surgery, surgical lengthenings of the rods are typically scheduled every four to six months depending on the individual's rate of growth. These lengthenings are performed in an operating room under general anesthesia. Small incisions are made to access the connectors between the rods. The rods are then manually elongated to lengthen the spine until resistance to further lengthening is encountered, typically after 6 to 10 mm (0.25 to 0.40 in) of lengthening. Each subsequent lengthening is done through the same small incisions. How much length is achieved depends on many factors, including how much the individual has grown between lengthenings and the flexibility of their spine. This procedure typically lasts about an hour and does not require an overnight stay in the hospital.

Magnetically controlled growing rods

Magnetically controlled growing rods (MCGRs) are adjustable metal rods that can be lengthened with a magnetic external remote control and are attached to the spine with screws or hooks (see Figure 4.4.2). They are inserted during a surgical procedure with limited fusions above and below the scoliosis curve, but unlike traditional growing rods that require repeat surgeries, MCGRs can be lengthened during routine clinical visits (see Figure 4.4.3), with the child being awake. While this visit may cause some children to feel nervous, it is a painless process.

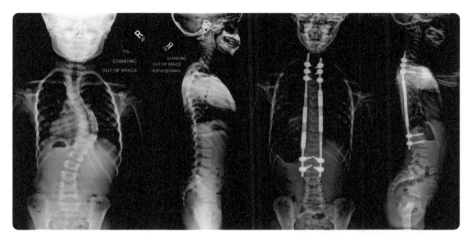

Figure 4.4.2 X-rays from before (left) and after (right) MCGR surgery.

MCGRs are, therefore, a noninvasive lengthening process that can reduce the burden of rod lengthenings and lower the overall treatment cost.[21] For example, an individual who has MCGR management may have as few as two surgeries for their scoliosis, while traditional growing rod treatment may require four or more surgeries. However, MCGR surgery may not be a suitable treatment method everywhere due to limited availability of the MCGR implant in some countries.[21]

The duration of the initial surgery varies but may take two to five hours. During this initial surgery, screws or hooks are attached to the vertebrae or ribs above and below the curve. Rods are attached to the screws or hooks and the spine is moved into a straighter position.

After implantation of MCGRs, individuals will recover in the hospital until they meet milestones required to be discharged and go home (see section 4.6). A typical length of time in the hospital is two days.

Regular follow-up for rod lengthening procedures occurs typically every two to three months depending on the individual's rate of growth. Typically, the rods are lengthened 2 to 4 mm (0.07 to 0.15 in) each visit.

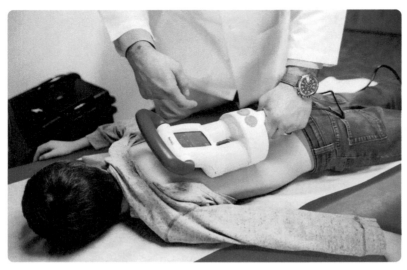

Figure 4.4.3 Lengthening of MCGRs. The child is placed on their stomach and the external remote control is used to lengthen the rods using magnetic force, which takes just one or two minutes.

Growth-friendly treatment surgical risks and long-term complications

Since growth-friendly treatment is not a single intervention, it might be thought of as a program, and over time this treatment is associated with a higher risk of complications for individuals with early-onset scoliosis (EOS).[14] Keep in mind that progressing scoliosis curves in a young, growing child itself presents greater risks. As such, the higher risk of surgery is acceptable as being necessary to provide maximum benefit for the individual.

Surgical risks for growth-friendly treatment include:

- **Neurologic injury:** There is a risk of neurologic injury (injury to the spinal cord or nerves resulting in temporary or permanent loss of function or sensation) during scoliosis surgery. During surgery, motor and sensory function* is carefully monitored in real time. This is referred to as "intraoperative neurophysiological monitoring"

---

* Motor function refers to the ability to move, while sensory function refers to the ability to receive and interpret information from the environment (e.g., vision, touch).

(IONM), or "intraoperative monitoring" (IOM). If any change in motor or sensory function is detected, the spine specialist immediately assesses the situation and takes appropriate action.

- **Postoperative infection:** There is a risk of infection after surgery, particularly infection of the surgical incisions. To decrease this risk, patients are instructed to wash with an antibacterial soap prior to surgery, surgery is performed using sterile techniques, and the patient receives IV antibiotics immediately before, during, and after surgery.

- **Excessive blood loss:** To decrease the risk of excessive blood loss, patients are given medication during surgery. At some hospitals, blood that is lost during surgery may be collected in a "cell saver." This collected blood can be concentrated and returned to the patient again if necessary. When necessary, donor blood transfusions may also be performed.

- **General anesthesia:** While general anesthesia is considered very safe, there are risks to its use. Most side effects are minor and temporary.[89] Risks include nausea, chills, vomiting, confusion, and a sore throat from the breathing tube used when a patient is under general anesthesia.[89] More information about general anesthesia risks is included in **Useful web resources**.

The following are potential long-term complications of growth-friendly treatment:

- **Pseudoarthrosis:** The failure of fusion; that is, the failure of the bones to unite properly. In growth-friendly treatment, pseudoarthrosis specifically refers to failure to fuse at the top and bottom anchor points of the instrumentation.

- **Instrumentation-related complications:** Loosening of implanted instrumentation, migration of instrumentation (shifting from intended location), or any other malfunction of instrumentation.

- **Proximal junctional kyphosis:** Hyperkyphosis that develops above the upper instrumented vertebra,*[91] which can weaken the connection between the screws and bone, causing the screws to pull out of the bone and/or for the instrumentation to be prominent (visible) through the skin.

---

* The "upper instrumented vertebra" is the highest vertebra (closest to the head) that is instrumented (has screws or hooks).

- **Development of additional spinal curvatures:** The development of additional curvatures above and below the surgical instrumentation (metal rods and screws or hooks); also referred to as "adding on."

The following summarizes what is known about the complications that may occur in each growth-friendly treatment type:

- **Traditional growing rods** require repeat surgeries to lengthen the rods, which increases the risk of complications. Complications occurred in 58 percent of individuals (all types of scoliosis), with an average of 2.2 complications per individual among those who reported complications.[94] The most common complications were instrumentation failure (screw/hooks failure, rod breakage) and infections.[94]
- **MCGR** treatment has similar but also unique complications compared to traditional growing rods. Complications occurred in 45 percent of individuals (all types of scoliosis).[95] The most commonly reported complications were unplanned revision surgery of the implants and instrumentation failure.[95] Additional complications include concern over metallosis (the buildup of metal debris in the soft tissues of the body), which has been observed in individuals with MCGRs, but the clinical consequences of this are unclear.[21] In 2020, the use of MCGRs (specifically the brand MAGnetic Expansion Control (MAGEC) by NuVasive Specialized Orthopedics) was suspended in the United Kingdom until the safety of this instrumentation could be confirmed.[96] As of February 2024, NuVasive Specialized Orthopedics has provided the Medicines and Healthcare products Regulatory Agency with enough safety reassurance for the suspension to be lifted.[96]

Next steps after growth-friendly treatment

Growth-friendly treatment has a finite timeline for effectively slowing the scoliosis progression. The average length of growth-friendly treatment for EOS is three to seven years.[21] There are many reasons that spine specialists may recommend ending growth-friendly treatment. Growth may slow or the spine may stiffen to the point where little length is gained. Alternatively, maximum length of the growing rods may be achieved, and/or the individual may reach adequate thoracic height of lung and chest development. When any of these milestones are reached, there are three main options:[21]

- Leave the instrumentation in the spine and monitor the individual.
- Remove the instrumentation in the spine and monitor the individual.
- Remove the instrumentation and perform a spinal fusion.

Of these options, removing instrumentation and having spinal fusion is the most common.[97] A spinal fusion following growth-friendly treatment allows for additional correction of the remaining scoliosis curve.[97] It is done most commonly between the ages of 11 and 13 years.[97]

Vertebral body tethering

Nothing is impossible, the word itself says "I'm possible"!
Audrey Hepburn

Vertebral body tethering (VBT) involves the surgical placement of screws in the vertebrae of the scoliosis curve through an anterior approach. The screws are placed on the convex side (outside) of the curve and then connected by a rope, referred to as a tether (Figure 4.5.1). The tension of the tether is strategically set to slow growth of the curve on the convex side, while enabling the spine to continue growing on the concave side (inside) of the scoliosis curve. As the individual grows, the spine begins to straighten. VBT is deemed a "growth harnessing" surgery, meaning that it uses the body's remaining growth as a force to gradually correct the scoliosis curve. This harnessing of growth to correct the scoliosis curve is referred to as "growth modulation."

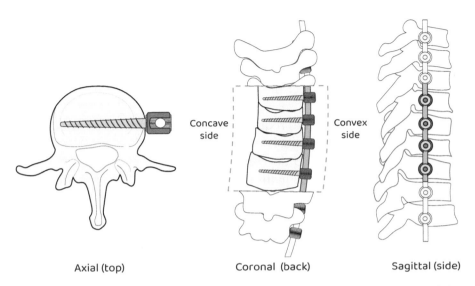

Concave side / Convex side

Axial (top)   Coronal (back)   Sagittal (side)

Figure 4.5.1 VBT instrumentation (screws with tether attached) in the spine: axial plane (left), coronal plane (middle), sagittal plane (right).

VBT goals

The primary goals of VBT are to:

- Stop curve progression
- Correct the spinal curve (decrease the Cobb angle)
- Maintain a balanced spine and posture
- Maintain spinal range of motion

Success for VBT is defined as a Cobb angle less than 35 degrees at the end of treatment and preventing the need for posterior spinal fusion. Sixty-eight percent of individuals with AIS had successful VBT treatment when assessed an average of 34 months after surgery.[98]

Who is a candidate for VBT?

The US Food and Drug Administration (FDA) has approved VBT* for use in individuals who meet the following criteria.[99]

- Skeletally immature and requiring surgical treatment to correct progressive idiopathic scoliosis
- Cobb angle of 30 to 65 degrees
- Bone tissue that is adequate to accommodate screw fixation (vertebrae have adequate size, shape, and density to handle insertion of screws)
- Have previously failed bracing (experienced significant curve progression while bracing) or been intolerant to brace wear

The following conditions are considered exclusion criteria for VBT, and this treatment should not be used in individuals who have any of these conditions:[99]

- An active infection—systemic infection, local infection, or skin compromise at the surgical site
- Prior spinal surgery on the same vertebrae
- Poor bone quality (defined as a T-score† of -1.5 or less)
- Skeletal maturity (defined as a Risser sign of 5 and a Sanders stage 8; see section 2.4)
- Underlying medical or surgical condition that precludes the potential benefit of spinal surgery (e.g., allergies to the implant materials)

These two lists are the widest possible criteria that individuals must satisfy to qualify for VBT. However, since the initial approval of VBT by the FDA, inclusion criteria have been an area of active research and

---

* The vertebral body tethering instrumentation used during VBT is classified as a Humanitarian Use Device (HUD) by the FDA. A HUD is defined as "a medical device intended to benefit patients in the treatment or diagnosis of a condition that affects or is manifested in not more than 8,000 individuals in the United States per year."[100] Traditional FDA approval for medical devices requires rigorous testing and research that may not be feasible to obtain when there are very few appropriate candidates for the device. The HUD designation indicates that the FDA has reviewed available safety information and determined that the tethering system likely provides benefits that outweigh the risks of its use. However, this device has not been studied using clinical trials and thus its long-term outcomes remain unknown.

† A T-score compares an individual's bone density with that of a typical, healthy young adult of the same gender. Negative T-scores indicate that an individual's bone density is below the average healthy adult's bone density.

controversy,[101,102] and specific criteria for VBT will vary among different medical centers and continue to evolve, such as limiting surgery to individuals who have a Cobb angle between 40 and 60 degrees instead of 30 to 65 degrees, and to individuals who are at specific stages of skeletal maturity (e.g., Risser 1 and Sanders 3). Because VBT relies on growth, the timing of this surgery with an individual's skeletal maturity is important. There are concerns that if VBT is performed too early, the scoliosis curve may overcorrect and begin to curve in the opposite direction.[101] Similarly, if VBT is performed too late, the individual may not have enough growth remaining to produce a lasting scoliosis correction.[101]

Tana

I specifically remember Lila had a hand X-ray that was used to determine her Sanders score (an indicator of how much skeletal growth she had remaining), which helped determine her surgical options. The doctor told us that we still had time before making any decisions, so we left that appointment with adjustments to her braces, a lot of information swirling through our minds, and many, many emotions.

As parents, we worried about how much of this information Lila understood, how much of this decision we were making for her, and how this would impact not only her physical health but also her mental health. These are very hard decisions for an adult, let alone a child.

My husband and I did our best to understand and explain Lila's condition and upcoming options and decisions to her. We do not work in medicine, so the only way we could begin to do this was to rely on Lila's wonderful care team providing us with information and allowing us to ask questions. They would encourage Lila to ask questions, too, but I could see the overwhelmed look on her face.

She later told us that she understood very little of what was being discussed that day. But what she did understand was the differences between the surgery options: that a spinal fusion had a more predictable outcome but may impact her movements and motion, while the tether surgery was a newer procedure, with a less predictable outcome, but one that would potentially allow her to continue doing all the activities that she loves with hopefully less impact to her motion. I think the decision to try the tether surgery was made as soon as we heard that. We understood that there were no guarantees, but we hoped that this would be the only surgery she needed.

Six months after learning that Lila would need surgery, we saw the doctor again for a regular follow-up appointment. Lila was 13 years old at the time. I had prepared myself before this appointment, but I was not prepared for the timing and urgency of the decisions about the surgery. Lila had continued to grow a little, but I was not expecting to hear that if we were going to elect to do the tether surgery, we should do so as soon as possible. This was in mid-November, and all I could think of was the holidays that were coming up. When would we fit this in? How could this very busy doctor fit this in?

The doctor casually suggested a date when he was scheduled for another VBT surgery, and therefore had a surgery team already lined up—in about five weeks. I remember him telling us something along the lines of his schedule being "irrelevant" when it comes to these surgeries; he would fit Lila in. I felt grateful!

In hindsight, I likely could have done a better job preparing Lila for these conversations and decisions. On our way home that day, she and I discussed what she understood from the appointment and what questions she had. A lot of her questions related to the surgery itself: Will I be awake? When will I be able to eat? When will I be able to go to the bathroom? Some I could answer, some I could not. Then I asked her a question; I wanted to know how she was feeling as she was not as emotional as she had been during her early brace appointments. She responded, "I feel great because everyone is doing everything they can to help me." I felt the same way and teared up hearing her gratitude and strength.

Lila

I had a tough decision to make: whether to have the surgery at all, and if so, which option. My parents and I decided that if I were to have surgery, the tether option was definitely right for me as it wouldn't limit my physical activity as much as a fusion would. We eventually scheduled a surgery date, and as the date got closer, I actually got very excited! After the surgery, I wouldn't have to wear either of my braces anymore, and after a short six weeks, I would be able to participate fully in activities again!

What happens during VBT?

VBT is performed in an operating room while the patient is under general anesthesia. The duration of the surgery varies but may take from three to five hours. During this surgery, the thoracic region of the spine is accessed through small ports inserted in the chest, between the ribs. To access the thoracic spine, one lung must be deflated. A general surgeon performs the small port access and helps the spine surgeon safely access the bones of the spine. The general surgeon may also help expose the lumbar spine through an incision along the side of the abdomen.

Screws are inserted into the vertebrae that make up the scoliosis curve, then the tether is attached to each screw and tightened while applying manual forces to reduce the curve. See Figure 4.5.2.

After the procedure is complete, the lung is reinflated and a tube is inserted into the chest (a chest tube) to remove excess air, drain any fluid that has accumulated in the chest, and promote expansion of the lung. This tube is typically left in for one or two days while the patient recovers in the hospital.

After VBT, individuals will stay in the hospital until they meet milestones required to be discharged and go home (see section 4.6). Typically, individuals are discharged after two days.

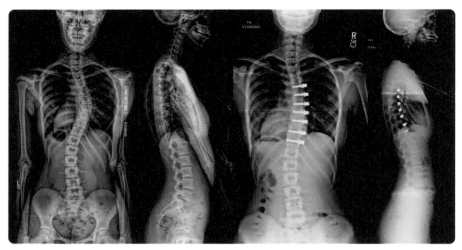

Figure 4.5.2 X-rays from before (left) and after (right) VBT. The tether is present connecting the screws but is made of a material that does not appear on the X-ray.

VBT surgical risks and long-term complications

The surgical risks for VBT include:

- **Neurologic injury:** There is a risk of neurologic injury (injury to the spinal cord or nerves resulting in temporary or permanent loss of function or sensation) during scoliosis surgery. During surgery, motor and sensory function* is carefully monitored in real time. This is referred to as "intraoperative neurophysiological monitoring" (IONM), or "intraoperative monitoring" (IOM). If any change in motor or sensory function is detected, the spine specialist immediately assesses the situation and takes appropriate action.
- **Postoperative infection:** There is a risk of infection after surgery, particularly infection of the surgical incision. To decrease this risk, patients are instructed to wash with an antibacterial soap prior to surgery, surgery is performed using sterile techniques, and the patient receives IV antibiotics immediately before, during, and after surgery.
- **Pulmonary complications:** These complications include pneumothorax (partial or complete lung collapse) and pleural effusion (excess

---

* Motor function refers to the ability to move, while sensory function refers to the ability to receive and interpret information from the environment (e.g., vision, touch).

collection of fluid surrounding the lungs). There is also a risk for bleeding around the lungs (hemothorax) in the days to weeks after surgery. The rate of pulmonary complications is 7 to 10 percent.[98,103]

- **Excessive blood loss:** To decrease the risk of excessive blood loss, patients are given medication during surgery. At some hospitals, blood that is lost during surgery may be collected in a "cell saver." This collected blood can be concentrated and returned to the patient if necessary. Also, when necessary, donor blood transfusions may be performed.

- **General anesthesia:** While general anesthesia is considered very safe, there are risks to its use. Most side effects are minor and temporary.[89] Risks include nausea, chills, vomiting, confusion, and a sore throat from the breathing tube used when a patient is under general anesthesia.[89] More information about general anesthesia risks is included in **Useful web resources.**

The following are potential long-term complications of VBT:

- **Tether breakage:** Tether breakage is the most common complication after VBT, affecting about 22 percent of individuals.[102,103] Typically, individuals are asymptomatic after tether breakage, and it has no impact on the spinal curve, but some individuals may lose correction.[102] Tether breakage is more common in individuals with lumbar curves than thoracic curves.[102]

- **Overcorrection:** The scoliosis curve may be overcorrected. The curve may straighten then begin to curve in the opposite direction of the initial curve. At an average of 34 months after surgery, overcorrection was observed in 11 to 14 percent of individuals.[98,103]

- **Development of additional spinal curvatures:** There is risk of developing additional curvature above and below the surgical instrumentation (metal rods and screws or hooks); also referred to as "adding on."

- **Instrumentation-related complications:** Implanted instrumentation may loosen, migrate (shift from intended location), or malfunction.

The overall complication rate in individuals with AIS who have VBT surgery is 23 to 28 percent at an average of two- to almost three-year follow-up.[98,93,103] Ideally, one VBT operation is the only surgery needed to correct an individual's scoliosis. However, complications of VBT can lead to a second surgery. This is called a reoperation and may include either a revision of the original tether or a conversion to a spinal fusion. The percentage of individuals undergoing reoperation increases with time, from 16 to 18 percent by three years[98,103] to 25 percent beyond three years.[93] Reoperation rates may continue to be higher as researchers follow individuals for longer times after surgery.

Spinal fusion versus VBT

Spinal fusion is the most common and predictable treatment for AIS. However, VBT has become increasingly popular.[98] Some of the initial appeal for VBT versus spinal fusion includes the potential for:

- Maintenance of spinal range of motion
- Maintenance of spine growth
- Less invasive surgery
- Quicker recovery and return to activities

However, because VBT is a fairly new surgery option, there are no long-term outcome studies to sufficiently address these potential benefits; only short-term outcomes are known. Additionally, it is not clear if the long-term efficacy of VBT (ability to correct the scoliosis curve) is comparable to a spinal fusion. There are no clinical trials to compare VBT with spinal fusion; thus, the evidence comparing the two surgeries is lacking and further research is required to assess if VBT is a superior approach to standard spinal fusion.[102]

Current research and understanding of the two treatments allows for the following comparisons in individuals with idiopathic scoliosis:

- **Curve correction:** Scoliosis curve correction in VBT is less reliable than spinal fusion[104] and less curve correction is obtained.[102] VBT does not provide as straight a spine as spinal fusion can, and it is common for individuals who undergo VBT to have a residual curve or rotation.
- **Complication rates:** Reported complication rates are significantly higher for VBT than for spinal fusion.[104] Individuals who have had VBT have a complication rate of 23 to 28 percent at an average follow-up of 24 to 34 months after surgery,[93,98,103] while individuals

who have had spinal fusion have a complication rate of 2 to 8 percent from time of surgery to an average follow-up of 47 months.[90,93]

- **Recovery time:** Individuals who undergo VBT have a shorter recovery time than individuals who undergo spinal fusion surgery.[102]
- **Spinal range of motion:** There is modest preservation of spinal range of motion with VBT,[104] greater than with spinal fusion.[102,105,106] However, experts question the significance of this motion for individuals and if it contributes to any meaningful impact on daily activities and sports participation.[61,106]
- **Spinal growth:** VBT is more likely to allow preserved spinal growth, while spinal fusion halts growth.[102] The exact amount of preserved spinal growth in comparison to spinal fusion is unclear.
- **Quality of life and functional outcomes:** Measures of quality of life and functional outcomes have been inconclusive with no difference observed between VBT and spinal fusion.[102,104,105]
- **Reoperation rates:** VBT is associated with a higher risk of reoperation.[104] At 36 months or more of follow-up, the reoperation rate for VBT is 25 percent compared to 2 percent for spinal fusion.[93]
- **Cost:** VBT is associated with higher costs than spinal fusion,[107] which may be an important consideration for families. Additionally, insurance companies may deny coverage for VBT, which means families may have to pay for all expenses.

Based on available research, it is believed that VBT holds promise as a scoliosis treatment method for specific curve types.[103,104] However, spinal fusion remains the most predictably successful treatment for thoracic curves in AIS, and more research about VBT is required.[102,104] It is important for families to be aware of the lack of research in this field. The "right" choice between VBT or spinal fusion will look different for each family. The spine specialist can help families establish treatment goals, balance their needs, and weigh the potential risks and benefits of each treatment accordingly.

Recovery after surgery

The greater the difficulty, the more the glory in surmounting it.

Epicurus

Common milestones that a patient must reach before they can leave the hospital after any of the three types of scoliosis surgeries discussed include being able to walk, tolerate food, urinate, and achieve reasonable pain control with pain medications that can be taken at home. A standard two-day recovery schedule after scoliosis surgery may look like the following:

- **Day of surgery:** The patient may experience drowsiness and/or dizziness when waking up from general anesthesia. They will be able to eat ice chips while their stomach wakes up and they eventually begin to take small sips of clear liquid. Pain control will be a focus after surgery, with pain medicine administered through an IV connected to a medicine pump. Patients should stand at the edge of the bed, with the assistance of care team members, on the evening of their surgery. At times this can be associated with light-headedness, nausea, or even vomiting.

- **Day one after surgery:** The patient will begin to mobilize (e.g., take steps). IV pain medication will be switched over to pain medication by mouth (orally). The urinary catheter will be removed. The patient will slowly start eating solid foods.
- **Day two after surgery:** The patient will continue to move around (e.g., walking and practicing stairs) so they feel prepared to move around at home. If the patient has not had a bowel movement yet and they have a history of constipation or are not tolerating food well, they may be given a suppository or enema (methods to help them have a bowel movement). Postoperative X-rays will be taken. The patient and family will receive any discharge medications and education materials about going home after surgery. Discharge paperwork will be signed and then the patient can leave the hospital.

Families are often concerned about pain after surgery. Pain is expected and is a normal part of healing. Pain is different for everyone, but patients often say the first three days at home are particularly challenging. Certain movements may be especially painful, and those movements may require assistance for a week or so. The individual may also have muscle spasms throughout the body that feel like squeezing pain and tightness. This can be improved by changing position, getting up and moving around, using heating pads, and/or taking medications. Pain can also make it difficult to sleep. Short naps during the day and changing positions frequently may help during the first few days after surgery.

At discharge, families may be sent home with narcotics (opioids) and muscle relaxants. It is expected that the individual will be slowly weaned off these medications and that they will be discontinued five to seven days after surgery. While narcotics are beneficial during this first week after surgery, they carry risks of dependence and addiction.[108] As such, spine specialists advise discontinuing these as soon as this can be safely accomplished. The use of over-the-counter pain medications such as acetaminophen (called paracetamol in some countries) may be continued for another two to three weeks as needed.

Note: Most spine specialists recommend *not* taking nonsteroidal anti-inflammatory drugs (NSAIDs, brand name: ibuprofen) after scoliosis fusion surgery as these medications have been shown to negatively impact and delay bone healing.[109]

Lila

A few days before the surgery, I started getting a bit nervous. There was a lot to do in preparation. I had to take a shower that night using a type of soap that smelled like a hospital. Then I had to do it again in the morning. Because I wasn't allowed to eat anything the morning of the surgery, the night before I ate three dinners!

When we got to the hospital, we checked in and all the prep began. Doctors started giving me IVs and, eventually, it was time to go into the operating room. I said goodbye to my parents and I was wheeled into a room where I was given medicine to keep me asleep and safe during surgery. I don't remember anything that happened during the surgery.

Tana

In preparation for the surgery, Lila had a few additional appointments. We scheduled a pre-op physical with her pediatrician. Gillette Children's also recommended that Lila meet with a counselor before her surgery to ask questions and discuss any worries or concerns. That appointment was over video chat, and it gave her a lot of reassurance on general questions relating to the hospital, surgery, and recovery. Lila also had an appointment with the pediatric general surgeon who would be assisting during the surgery.

Once we arrived at the hospital and Lila's name was called from the waiting room, we went to a room with a hospital bed and two chairs and waited. On the bed was a purple blanket made and donated by volunteers that was a gift for Lila; this made her smile. Lila changed into a hospital gown, and nurses came in to prepare her for surgery. Numerous nurses and doctors stopped in to talk to us, which was a nice distraction and made the time pass quicker. Before they wheeled her into the operating room, we hugged her and told her we would see her soon.

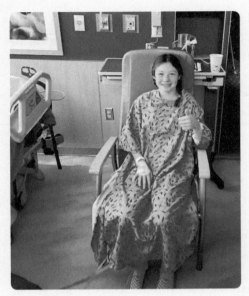

Lila in the hospital the morning after her surgery.

Lila

When I woke up from surgery, I felt a little bit lost and confused, but when I saw my parents, I remembered why I was at the hospital. I remember a lot of tubes connected to me and some machines behind me, but my memory of this time is a bit messed up. My parents have some stories of what I said while I was like this. One of them is that when the nurse came to check on me in the middle of the night, I told her that I wanted to be a nurse and help people like she does. I don't remember saying that and I am not sure that I want to be a nurse, but it seems like a nice thing to say to someone who is helping you out.

I also had a catheter tube for a while, but eventually they removed it and I had to start getting up to use the toilet. I was told that before I could leave the hospital, I had to complete some tests: just walking, walking up and down stairs, going to the toilet, and a few other things.

Once I was back home, I sat on the couch a lot watching *Friends* on TV. Something kind of interesting that I noticed was a weird tingly sensation at the bottom of my ribs on the left side. I thought it was cool, but I realized the area around the tingly part was numb and I couldn't feel anything there. My mom marked the numb area with a pen so I could see if it would shrink or get bigger. Now that area is much smaller but still a little numb, and I still cannot feel things there like I can in other areas on my stomach.

Tana

We were told that Lila's surgery would take two and a half to three hours, but in less than two hours, the doctor was in the waiting room to tell us that the surgery went great. He also gave us a piece of the tether that they used on her spine to show her. We were able to see her about 45 minutes later in the post-op area.

Later, while she was still in the hospital, they did an X-ray of her spine, and looking at it we could see the tether and screws in her spine, and that immediately her curve was improved.

When we first saw Lila after the surgery, she was covered in blankets from head to toe. The only thing we could see was her face sticking out of an oval hole in the blankets. She briefly woke up and smiled at us. It was a great relief seeing her beautiful face and eyes open! For the next hour, she was in and out of sleep, and not making much sense when she was awake. The whole time a nurse consistently came in to check on her.

Lila spent about 48 hours in the hospital following her surgery. I stayed with her through the first night, and her dad stayed with her the second night. She was in a comfortable room with plenty of space around her bed, a couch for mom or dad, and a large bathroom.

Lila was restless the first night, and while the pain medications made her comfortable, they also made her emotional. She would sleep for about an hour at a time, and when she woke up, she would be crying and upset but couldn't articulate what was wrong. When I later asked her, she said she has no memory of this. She was hungry soon after surgery, but because she was drowsy from medications, she could only make it through a few bites at a time.

She had a chest tube connected to her following the surgery (this is specific to individuals who undergo VBT) until a couple of hours before we left the hospital. She said the chest tube didn't hurt, but made it difficult to get comfortable. She also had a catheter in through the first night. Once they took out the catheter, she then had to manage her way to the bathroom with her IV and chest tube still connected. By the next day, they had her sitting up in a chair.

After the second night in the hospital, we were told that Lila could go home after certain tasks were completed, such as the thoracic doctor approving the chest tube coming out, and Lila walking a flight of stairs. They gave her some pain medications shortly before we were leaving to help keep her comfortable on the drive home. I'm sure the medicines helped, but Lila was not comfortable during that car ride (she also has no memory of this, either).

Once home, Lila slept a lot the first two days, and I slept on the floor in her room the first few nights. The doctor prescribed both pain medication and muscle relaxers to keep her comfortable. The medication schedule was a bit overwhelming in the first few days, so we tracked each dose in writing. Lila soon discovered that she did not like taking the pain medication as it made her feel disoriented and she had a difficult time remembering things. Within a few days, we weaned her off the pain medication, but she continued to take the muscle relaxers for about a week to help stay comfortable.

Following surgery, temporary restrictions to movement and activity are required to help the body heal. These are detailed for each surgery type in Table 4.6.1. It is important to follow the timeline the spine specialist recommends. It is often helpful to work with school staff (e.g., teachers, school counselor, gym teacher) to facilitate a safe return to school and eventually other school activities such as gym class.

Table 4.6.1 Typical recovery timeline after scoliosis surgery

RECOVERY MILESTONE	SPINAL FUSION	GROWTH-FRIENDLY	VBT
Discontinue prescription pain medication	5 to 7 days	5 to 7 days	5 to 7 days
Return to school (half days)	1 to 2 weeks	1 to 2 weeks	1 to 2 weeks
Return to school (full days)	3 weeks	3 weeks	3 weeks
Able to fully submerge surgical incision	6 weeks	6 weeks	6 weeks
Return to light activity (e.g., biking or using an elliptical machine)	6 weeks	6 weeks	6 weeks
Clearance for activities including running, jumping, bending, twisting, or lifting more than 5 to 10 lb (2 to 5 kg)	3 months	3 months	6 weeks
Return to full activity including sports	3 to 6 months	3 to 6 months	6 to 8 weeks depending on activity*

* Clearance for sports that are considered collision sports (e.g., American football, ice hockey, rugby) may take longer than clearance for minimal or noncontact sports (e.g., volleyball, baseball, gymnastics).

Families often wonder what will happen to the spinal instrumentation (rods/tether and screws or hooks) in the individual's back after spinal fusion or VBT surgery. For most individuals, this instrumentation will remain in their back for the rest of their life without issue. In later years, if problems arise with the instrumentation, it is possible to have some or all of it removed, but it is very uncommon to remove spine instrumentation. Another common question families ask about their spine instrumentation is if it will trigger metal detectors. It will not.

Lila

I'm happy I had the tether surgery. I think it was a great option for me because of all the activities I enjoy doing. I also think the recovery was pretty quick: I was able to get off many of the medications much quicker than they thought. The doctors were really nice and helpful during my recovery, and I am glad I no longer have to wear my braces at night or during the day. My back no longer limits my everyday activities, and it rarely hurts.

I've been surprised by how much I've grown since the surgery! I came out of surgery immediately taller and have grown another 3 inches (7.6 cm) since then.

Now more than a year after the tether surgery, I feel great. To someone considering scoliosis surgery, I would say that it is worth it because it will help your back and you will be able to still do all sorts of fun activities after your recovery. The only times I remember it hurting was right after the surgery, especially if I was lying in a weird position, and occasionally for a few weeks after surgery.

Sometimes I worry that the curves in my back will worsen and I will have to have another surgery or be put in a brace again, but then I remember that I'm at a really good hospital with great doctors and that if I need further care, they will take care of me and I have no need to worry.

Tana

About two weeks after Lila's surgery, we had a family get-together for the holidays, and everyone commented that she appeared completely normal and they would have never known she had just had surgery. About three weeks after surgery, she returned to school.

Lila had some restrictions for the first six weeks, including no twisting, bending, or lifting anything over 10 lb (4.5 kg). That meant she couldn't initially wear her backpack to school as it was too heavy. So while she felt she drew less attention without her brace, she did draw some attention and questions because she had to carry her notes and iPad in a zipped binder instead of a backpack.

Lila didn't have any pain during this time but had to work very hard to be mindful to only do things within the restrictions. She was thrilled when the doctor lifted the restrictions after six weeks, telling her she could gradually return to activities and sports. At that appointment, she measured about a half inch (1.3 cm) taller. Her X-rays also showed about a 20-degree improvement in her curve (about 50 percent straighter).

Three months after surgery, Lila was back to running and playing soccer. At four months, she went surfing. Five months after surgery, she was hiking and riding horseback in the mountains. We were thrilled with her quick healing and ability to participate in all these activities and adventures!

It's now about 19 months post-surgery. Lila has grown nearly 3 inches (7.6 cm), her tether was still in place as of her last appointment two months ago, and her curve has remained in a range the doctor likes (about 20 degrees less than it was before surgery). We are so happy with the decision for Lila to have the tether surgery and grateful for the opportunity!

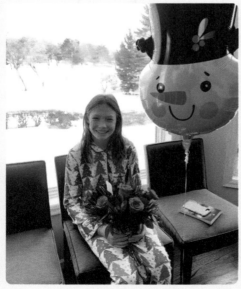

Lila at home three days after VBT surgery.

Follow-up visits after surgery

After surgery, follow-up visits with a spine specialist will be required at specific intervals based on the surgery type. A typical timeline is:

- **Spinal fusion:** 6 weeks, 6 months, and 12 months after surgery
- **Growth-friendly treatment:** 6 weeks and 3 months after surgery and regular lengthening visits as needed based on type of growth-friendly treatment
- **VBT:** Every 4 to 6 months until skeletal maturity

Halo gravity traction

Do the difficult things while they are easy and do the great things while they are small. A journey of a thousand miles must begin with a single step.

Lao Tzu

Halo gravity traction is a multistage treatment for severe scoliosis to stretch and straighten the spine and soft tissues (skin, muscle, ligaments) prior to scoliosis surgery.

A metal ring (halo) is surgically attached to the outer surface of the individual's skull bone using small metal pins (Figure 4.7.1). The ring is then connected to a pulley system that applies a force (traction), pulling the head and spine upward. Over the course of treatment (three to six weeks or longer, depending on the treatment center), the pulling force is increased. The individual stays in hospital for the entire duration of their halo gravity traction treatment and frequent skin checks and neurologic exams are required.

The goals of halo traction are to slowly stretch the spine, soft tissues (skin, muscles, ligaments), and spinal cord to reduce neurological risk during surgery; maximize curve correction; and improve pulmonary function before scoliosis surgery.[110,111]

Halo gravity traction may be recommended to individuals who meet either of the following criteria:

- Cobb angle greater than 100 degrees
- Concurrent hyperkyphosis

Criteria may be different depending on the medical center.

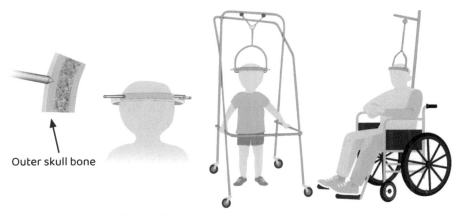

Outer skull bone

Figure 4.7.1 Halo gravity traction.

The metal ring is attached to the skull using 4 to 12 small pins in an operating room while the patient is under general anesthesia. The procedure typically takes only 20 to 30 minutes.

During the hospital stay, the individual's neurologic status, including movement and strength, will be checked daily, and the pins will be cleaned to prevent infection of the pin sites. X-rays of the spine will be taken weekly to monitor progress. More information is included in **Useful web resources.**

There are potential risks to halo gravity traction. These include but are not limited to:[112]

- Neck pain
- Pin loosening
- Pin site skin infections
- Neurologic changes

The overall complication rate for both idiopathic and nonidiopathic scoliosis ranges from 17 to 38 percent,[113,114,115,116] with one study of idiopathic scoliosis patients reporting temporary and minor complications in 95 percent of individuals.[112] It is important to recall that individuals being treated with halo gravity traction are those with the worst curvatures undergoing the highest risk procedures due to the severity of their spinal curve.

Halo gravity traction treatment ends when the final pulling force is reached and satisfactory curve improvement has been achieved. The individual will then proceed to their scoliosis surgery and their halo will be removed. Scoliosis surgery and halo removal typically happen within the same surgery. After halo removal, the individual may be prescribed a temporary neck brace to help with comfort and support.

Key points Chapter 4

- The overall goals of scoliosis surgery are to stop curve progression, improve the spinal curve, and achieve a balanced spine and posture.
- All surgical procedures have potential risks and complications.
- Spinal fusion is the most common type of scoliosis surgery. It involves fusing (joining together) two or more vertebrae in the spine. Typically, metal rods and screws (termed "instrumentation" or "implants") are used to hold the spine in the straighter position and facilitate fusion between the bones.
- Spinal fusion halts the growth of the spine and is generally not appropriate for very young children.
- Growth-friendly treatment refers to treatment that places surgical instrumentation (metal rods and screws or hooks) in the spine without fusing (permanently joining together) the vertebrae or with limited fusion. The length of the metal rods can be expanded over time to limit curve progression or partially correct curves while allowing a young child to continue to grow.
- Traditional growing rods are manually lengthened during surgical procedures under general anesthesia.
- Magnetically controlled growing rods (MCGRs) are lengthened via a magnetic remote control in clinic.
- Removal of instrumentation and conversion to spinal fusion is the most common next step following the end of growth-friendly treatment.
- Vertebral body tethering (VBT) involves the surgical placement of screws in the vertebrae and is a fairly new surgery option. The screws are placed on the convex side (outside) of the curve and then connected by a rope, referred to as a tether.
- Spinal fusion is the most common and predictable treatment for AIS, however VBT has become increasingly popular for the following potential benefits: maintenance of spinal range of motion, maintenance of spine growth, less invasive surgery, and quicker recovery and return to activities.
- Reported complication rates are significantly higher for VBT than they are for spinal fusion.

Chapter 5

The adult with idiopathic scoliosis

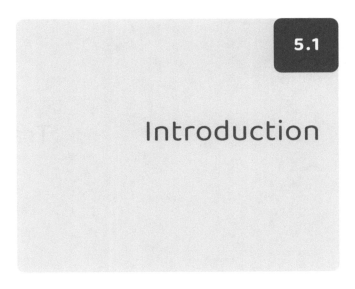

Introduction

5.1

> The little reed, bending to the force of the wind,
> soon stood upright again when the storm had passed over.
>
> **Aesop**

In most cases, an individual will have a mild curve (less than 35 degrees) at the time of skeletal maturity. For these mild curves, routine check-ins with a spine specialist are not necessary in adulthood. Those with more moderate curves (35 to 49 degrees), may be recommended to transition to adult care once they are skeletally mature. This typically involves establishing check-ins with a primary care provider or, depending on curve size and prior treatment, with an adult spine specialist. For individuals who enter adulthood with a Cobb angle of 50 degrees or greater, it is highly recommended that they establish care with a spine specialist and undergo surgery for their scoliosis.

USEFUL WEB RESOURCES

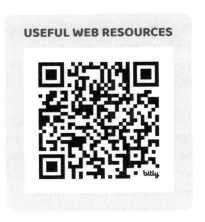

Transition to adult care

Things which matter most must never be
at the mercy of things which matter least.
Goethe

Health care transition is defined as the planned process and skill-building to empower adolescents and their families to navigate an adult model of health care. It is more than just changing medical professionals (simply termed "transfer").

Pediatric services for scoliosis care are usually much better resourced and are more proactive in following up with the individual than are adult services. With adult services for scoliosis care, it is usually up to the individual and family to find new services and providers.

Transition involves three steps: preparing for, transferring to, and integrating into adult services. Figure 5.2.1 shows a typical form that can be used for the first step—preparing an individual for transition to adult services. Note that just because a file has been transferred over does not mean that the individual has successfully integrated into an adult service provider.

Transition Readiness Assessment Questionnaire (TRAQ)

Patient Name: _____   Date of Birth: ___/___/___Today's Date ___/___/___ (MRN#_____)

Directions to Youth and Young Adults: Please check the box that best describes *your* skill level in the following areas that are important for transition to adult health care. There is no right or wrong answer and your answers will remain confidential and private.
Directions to Caregivers/Parents: If your youth or young adult is unable to complete the tasks below on their own, please check the box that best describes *your* skill level. **Check here** if you are a parent/caregiver completing this form. ☐

	No, I do not know how	No, but I want to learn	No, but I am learning to do this	Yes, I have started doing this	Yes, I always do this when I need to
Managing Medications					
1. Do you fill a prescription if you need to?					
2. Do you know what to do if you are having a bad reaction to your medications?					
3. Do you reorder medications before they run out?					
4. Do you explain any medications (name and dose) you are taking to healthcare providers?					
5. Do you speak with the pharmacist about drug interactions or other concerns related to your medications?					
Appointment Keeping					
6. Do you call the doctor's office to make an appointment?					
7. Do you follow-up on referrals for tests or check-ups or labs?					
8. Do you arrange for your ride to medical appointments?					
9. Do you call the doctor about unusual changes in your health (for example: allergic reactions)?					
Tracking Health Issues					
10. Do you fill out the medical history form, including a list of your allergies?					
11. Do you keep a calendar or list of medical and other appointments?					
12. Do you tell the doctor or nurse what you are feeling?					
13. Do you contact the doctor when you have a health concern?					
14. Do you make or help make medical decisions pertaining to your health?					
15. Do you attend your medical appointment or part of your appointment by yourself?					
Talking with Providers					
16. Do you ask questions of your nurse or doctor about your health or health care?					
17. Do you answer questions that are asked by the doctor, nurse, or clinic staff?					
18. Do you ask your doctor or nurse to explain things more clearly if you do not understand their instructions to you?					
19. Do you tell the doctor or nurse whether you followed their advice or recommendations?					
20. Do you explain your health history to your healthcare providers (including past surgeries, allergies, and medications)?					

Please circle how you feel about the following statements	Not at all important	Not too important	Somewhat important	Important	Very Important
How important is it to you to manage your own health care?	1	2	3	4	5
How confident do you feel about your ability to manage your own health care?	1	2	3	4	5

© Wood, Reiss, & Livingood, McBee, Johnson, 2020

Figure 5.2.1 Transition Readiness Assessment Questionnaire. Reproduced with kind permission from Dr. David L. Wood.

The following are some pointers on transition for an individual with scoliosis:

- Get help from the pediatric scoliosis care team (and possibly others) as to who would be the best adult health professional based on your scoliosis treatment history.
- Make a summary of the scoliosis and your relevant medical history with someone who knows your experience, such as your parent or health professional. When meeting new health professionals, it is helpful to have a short (one- to two-minute) summary of the health care journey to date that can help guide the conversation, or, if easier, a one-page written summary you have prepared to hand to a new health professional. This summary should include the type of scoliosis, history of treatments, and current challenges. This information will be very helpful to the new adult health professional.
- Consider gathering all relevant surgical reports and imaging that have been performed for future reference. Recent clinical notes may also be helpful.
- Be open and honest with new health professionals. You are the expert on your own health. The more information given to the care team, the better they can meet any needs.
- Don't wait and see. If any changes in the spine occur or any problems arise (such as persistent pain); visit a primary care provider or a spine specialist for advice.
- Be prepared to advocate for any medical needs that can give you more control over quality of life. Remember to stay calm and polite but assertive to get the support or information needed.

Got Transition is a US federally funded national resource center for health care transition. Its aim is to improve transition from pediatric to adult health care using evidence-based strategies for health professionals, adolescents, young adults, and their families. The website has a lot of useful guidance and is included in **Useful web resources**.

Adulthood with idiopathic scoliosis

For in every adult there dwells the child that was, and in every child there lies the adult that will be.

John Connolly

At some point in the scoliosis journey, individuals with idiopathic scoliosis and their families start to wonder how their diagnosis will affect their future adult life. This section addresses common concerns individuals and families have about adulthood for individuals with idiopathic scoliosis.

Spine specialist follow-up

As noted above, in most cases an individual will have a mild curve (less than 35 degrees) at the time of skeletal maturity. For these mild curves, routine check-ins with a spine specialist are not necessary in adulthood. Those with more moderate curves (35 to 49 degrees) may be recommended to transition to adult care once they are skeletally mature.

It is possible for idiopathic curves to progress during adulthood, but the progression is usually very slow.[3] The risk of scoliosis progression after skeletal maturity increases with curve size.

Following up with a spine specialist is recommended for all individuals with scoliosis if spine-related symptoms arise, such as signs of scoliosis progression, loss of height, or persistent back pain.

The following criteria provide a general guideline for counseling individuals on spine follow-up in adulthood. These criteria may vary among medical centers:

- **Individuals who have had surgery:** Once individuals have completed standard post-surgery follow-up, routine spine specialist follow-up is not necessary.
- **Nonsurgically treated individuals with a Cobb angle less than 35 degrees:** Routine follow-up with a spine specialist is not necessary after ending pediatric care.
- **Nonsurgically treated individuals with a Cobb angle of 35 to 49 degrees:** Individuals should have X-rays taken every two to five years. These can be taken with a primary care provider. If several X-rays over time indicate that the curve has not progressed, this observation may be discontinued. However, if X-rays demonstrate curve progression or if new back-related symptoms arise, it is recommended that these individuals re-establish care with an adult spine specialist for further examination.
- **Nonsurgically treated individuals with a Cobb angle of 50 degrees or greater:** It is highly recommended that individuals with a Cobb angle of 50 degrees or greater have surgery. If the individual decides not to pursue surgical intervention, spine specialists may recommend X-rays be taken and reviewed every one to two years until age 25. If these X-rays confirm the scoliosis curve is stable (not increasing), then further X-rays are recommended only if new symptoms arise. If the scoliosis curve continues to progress, it is recommended that the individual reconsider surgery. As the curve continues to progress, surgical options become more limited and have higher complications rates. A curve may reach a size where the risks of surgery outweigh the benefits, and spine specialists will no longer consider surgical intervention. Living with large and progressive curves can

also lead to a decrease in quality of life (increased pain, limited function, difficulty breathing).

Natural aging of the spine

As an individual gets older, changes occur to the spine as part of the normal aging process. This applies to the general population as well as to people with idiopathic scoliosis. This aging process is variable across people in rate and extent, resulting in variable clinical impact.

Age-related changes in the general population without scoliosis or major medical conditions can include:[117]

- **Disc degeneration:** a breakdown and thinning of the intervertebral discs
- **Osteoarthritis:** cartilage breakdown in the facet joints of the spine
- **Surrounding ligament and muscle changes:** ligament shortening and loss of flexibility; loss of muscle mass
- **Osteoporosis:** a loss in bone density that is significantly lower than typical for a person's age
- **Osteopenia:** bone density that is not typical but not as low as osteoporosis

In the general population, these degenerative changes in the intervertebral discs, facet joints, ligaments, and muscles can cause back pain that is specific to the lower back or pain that radiates throughout the body.[117]

Individuals with idiopathic scoliosis may experience higher rates of degenerative changes than those in the general population. The specific treatments an individual has had also impacts the degree of degenerative changes. Degenerative changes include:

- **Disc degeneration:** A higher level of degenerative disc changes occurs in individuals who received surgical or bracing treatment.[118] A known complication of spinal fusion is accelerated degeneration of the cartilage and intervertebral discs in the adjacent nonoperated vertebrae, referred to as "adjacent segment disease."[29] Adjacent segment disease is far more common in spinal fusions that extend into the lower lumbar spine than in those that end in the lower thoracic or upper lumbar spine.

- **Osteoarthritis:** A higher severity of osteoarthritis in facet joints occurs in individuals with adolescent idiopathic scoliosis (AIS) than individuals without scoliosis.[119]
- **Osteoporosis:** Individuals with idiopathic scoliosis have a lower bone density throughout their body than the general population and display an increased prevalence of osteopenia and osteoporosis.[39] The reason for this is still unclear.

Individuals can try to maintain bone density as they age by taking supplements and following these lifestyle recommendations:

- **Eat foods that support bone health:** Prioritize getting adequate calcium, vitamin D, and protein through diet or supplements[120] (e.g., dairy products, leafy green vegetables, egg yolks).
- **Stay active:** Do weight-bearing exercise such as strength training, walking, hiking, or jogging,[120] as well as core (abdominal and back) strengthening activities.
- **Avoid smoking and other nicotine products:** Cigarette smoking is significantly associated with reduced bone density.[121] Research on other nicotine products such as e-cigarettes is limited but suggests that nicotine may negatively impact the viability and function of bone cells.[121]
- **Limit alcohol intake:** Excessive alcohol can harm bones.[120]

Health-related quality of life

Current long-term outcomes research indicates that most individuals treated for idiopathic scoliosis (by observation, bracing, and/or surgery) typically live healthy and active adult lives relatively unaffected by their condition.

Health-related quality of life (HRQOL) is defined as "an individual's or a group's perceived physical and mental health over time."[68] The HRQOL for individuals with scoliosis is typically assessed through standardized questionnaires. These include the Scoliosis Research Society Instrument 22-R (SRS-22r), a scoliosis-specific questionnaire on pain, function, self-image, mental health, and satisfaction with care.[122] There are other non-scoliosis-specific questionnaires that contain similar questions.

HRQOL findings related to physical activity, physical function, pain, and mental and social health include:

- **Physical activity** (participation in sports or exercise): Individuals who received treatment for juvenile idiopathic scoliosis (JIS) or AIS have a level of physical activity in adulthood comparable to the general population when assessed 19 years after surgery and 27 years after ending brace treatment.[123] Age of onset (JIS versus AIS) did not have an impact on level of physical activity.[123]
- **Physical function** (performing activities of daily living): Individuals who received treatment (spinal fusion or bracing) for JIS or AIS report a slightly lower level of overall physical function than the general population 10 to 20 years after completion of treatment.[124,125]
- **Lung function:** Individuals with AIS who had either been treated surgically or with bracing had improved pulmonary (lung) function 1.5 and 25 years after treatment.[126]
- **Pain:** Individuals who received treatment (spinal fusion or bracing) for their AIS report slightly higher levels of general bodily pain, neck pain, and back pain than the general population 20 years after treatment.[124,127] This pain does not typically compromise level of activity or ability to work, and it is believed to be much less than that experienced by individuals with large, untreated scoliosis curves.
- **Mental and social health:** Psychological well-being in individuals with AIS who received surgery (spinal fusion) or brace treatment is comparable to the general population at an average of 20 years after completion of treatment.[124]

Pregnancy and childbirth

Individuals with idiopathic scoliosis and their families often worry about the long-term effects of idiopathic scoliosis on pregnancy and childbirth. While research is limited and unclear, most women with scoliosis can conceive, carry, and deliver healthy babies without significant changes in their care or increased risk to themselves or their baby. If the individual or their obstetrician has any concerns on how scoliosis may impact pregnancy or delivery, it is recommended that an adult spine specialist be consulted to evaluate the individual's specific risk profile. The following summarizes what current research suggests about various factors in pregnancy and childbirth:

- **Success of pregnancy:** Regardless of treatment type, women with AIS typically have a similar number of children as the general population. Some studies suggest that women with AIS may be slightly less likely to become pregnant and slightly more likely to seek fertility treatment than the general population. However, research has not demonstrated any direct connection between AIS and infertility, and the relationship between these two is not understood.[128]
- **Age at pregnancy and duration:** There does not appear to be any difference in the age at which women with AIS conceive or their rate of full-term or premature births.[128]
- **Curve progression during pregnancy:** There appears to be no difference in curve progression during pregnancy in women who have had surgical treatment for AIS compared to those who have not been pregnant.[129]
- **Back pain during pregnancy:** Women with AIS experience slightly higher rates of back pain during pregnancy than pregnant peers in the general population. This back pain is reported as not debilitating, and it resolves after delivery.[128] Furthermore, the incidence of back pain may be higher only in women with AIS who have had spinal fusion that extends to their third or fourth lumbar vertebra (L3 or L4).[130]
- **Delivery complications:** Studies show that women with AIS experience similar rates of cesarean delivery (C-section) as the general population.[128] Women with AIS treated surgically with spinal fusion have C-sections more frequently than women in the general population.[130,131]
- **Epidural placement:** Women with AIS who have received surgical treatment, specifically spinal fusion, can still have an epidural placed during delivery, but there is an increased risk of minor, but reversible, complications.[128] Women who did not receive surgical treatment for scoliosis have comparable epidural experiences compared to peers in general population.

Key points Chapter 5

- In most cases, an individual will have a mild curve (less than 35 degrees) at the time of skeletal maturity. For these mild curves, routine check-ins with a spine specialist are not necessary in adulthood.

- Individuals with more moderate curves (35 to 49 degrees), may be recommended to transition to adult care once they are skeletally mature.

- It is highly recommended that individuals with a Cobb angle of 50 degrees or greater undergo surgery. Skeletally mature individuals who have not received surgical treatment for their scoliosis with a Cobb angle of 50 degrees or greater are at higher risk of curve progression throughout adulthood.

- Health care transition is the planned process and skill-building to empower adolescents and their families to navigate an adult model of health care.

- Pediatric services for scoliosis care are usually much better resourced and are more proactive in following up with the individual than adult services.

- Following up with a spine specialist is recommended for all individuals with scoliosis if spine-related symptoms arise, such as signs of scoliosis progression, loss of height, or persistent back pain.

- Individuals with idiopathic scoliosis may experience higher rates of degenerative changes in the spine than individuals in the general population.

- Most individuals treated for idiopathic scoliosis (by observation, bracing, and/or surgery) typically live healthy and active adult lives relatively unaffected by their condition.

- Most women with scoliosis can conceive, carry, and deliver healthy babies without significant changes in their care or increased risk to mother or baby.

Chapter 6

Living with idiopathic scoliosis

> What lies behind us and what lies before us
> are tiny matters compared to what lies within us.
> **Oliver Wendell Holmes**

In this chapter, people share stories of living with idiopathic scoliosis.

Brett and Lindsey, parents of six-year-old Andrew, with infantile idiopathic scoliosis (IIS), from Minnesota, US

As a baby, Andrew was joyful, healthy, and relaxed—easy compared to his big brother—and he was meeting developmental milestones. When he was about seven months old, we noticed he favored his left side and often propped himself up on his left elbow. When rolling from tummy to back, he only ever rolled one way, and in the high chair, he predominantly used his left hand. At his nine-month appointment, the pediatrician ordered X-rays and made a referral to a pediatric orthopedic spine specialist.

On April 23, 2018, the day before Andrew turned 10 months old, we received a diagnosis of progressive infantile idiopathic scoliosis. His supine (lying down, face up) X-ray showed his spine had a curve of 65 degrees and a rib vertebral angle difference (RVAD) of 40 degrees, a significant curve that's compounded by a twisting of the spine. A curvature of 70 to 80 degrees begins to impair lung and organ development and function, so we were told that swift medical intervention was required to minimize and hopefully correct the impact.

The diagnosis was frightening and completely turned our world upside down. Our healthy and happy baby suddenly needed the urgent attention of specialists. We were filled with fear and consumed by what this meant for our son's future. We scoured the Internet for resources and information about children who have had this diagnosis and were left with few beneficial resources and many scary stories. Later, we discovered a community on social media that quickly became our trusted source for information and ideas, outlet for frustration, and giver of endless support.

Our doctors advised us that we should move to Mehta casting as soon as possible. Because Andrew was approaching his first birthday, we were acutely aware that our window for a potential cure was closing quickly. We agreed that casting would be the best nonsurgical option.

Andrew got his first cast on May 15 and was fussy and frustrated with it for about a week. He couldn't move around like he was used to, the bulk of his cast kept him from reaching and even seeing most of the food on his high chair tray, his tiny arms couldn't reach what he wanted, he couldn't find a comfortable seated position while on the floor, and it was impossible for him to get back up to a seated position from lying down. But he showed incredible resiliency and persistence, and within a week he'd figured out how to maneuver in a comfortable way.

Over the next 18 months, Andrew had five different casts, each one lasting between 6 and 12 weeks. We had several setbacks and scheduled breaks along the way, including one casting that had to be postponed because Andrew spiked a fever, but through it all, his curve continued to decrease.

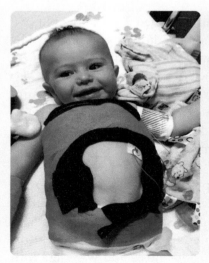 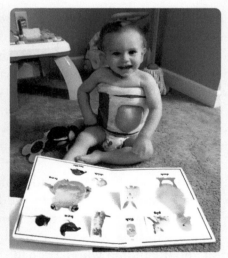

Andrew in two different casts during casting treatment.

Having a casted baby brought about a whole new spectrum of challenges: The quantity of food he ate decreased dramatically, as the rigid cast restricted his stomach. Smaller frequent snacks became the norm. He lost some of his adorable baby chubbiness, and it was replaced with chiseled baby muscle from constantly hauling around a cast that weighed 20 percent of his own body weight.

Every crumb, noodle, grain, or drip had the chance of making its way down into the torso of his cast, which could lead to skin irritation, sores, and even ulcers. We quickly moved from using bibs to children's art smocks during mealtime.

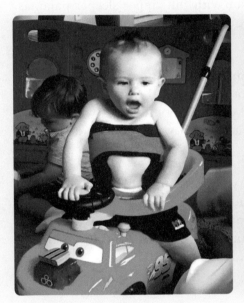 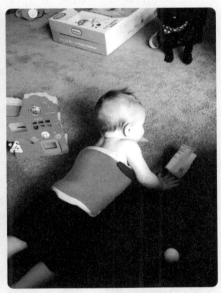

Andrew playing in his cast.

Each diaper change held the possibility of a blowout. Since bathtime wasn't an option, frequent changes were necessary. We experimented with several different diaper brands and found one that worked best for Andrew's specific casts; the design was very high on the backside so we could tuck it between the cast and his lower back. And when blowouts happened (and they definitely did happen), we learned the power of using just a tiny bit of witch hazel to remove the urine-soaked moleskin smell from the cast.

Keeping Andrew's body temperature regulated was a struggle. We were told to expect him to get warm and overheat easily, but I didn't expect that would mean he would be sleeping in an air-conditioned house in just his diaper.

Messy play, finger painting, gardening, water play, sandboxes, sticky Popsicles, Play-Doh, bath time, and swimming were simply off the table. Having a child in a cast during the precious summer months of Minnesota was so frustrating.

Dressing him took some creativity. We found that the easiest way to clothe Andrew was with rompers or with full zipper sleeper pajamas. Anything with a waistband was out of the question with the fit of Andrew's cast.

Well-meaning strangers made comments about how big Andrew was, and on occasion, people we did not know would reach out and touch him. I know many people were just curious about what it was that was making him look so big and awkward, but it was an odd and irritating experience.

Following his fifth cast, Andrew's stubborn curve plateaued and was no longer responding. Under the advice of our doctors, we moved to bracing, which felt like a huge defeat. We were told that it was unlikely that bracing would provide continued improvement, and the goal now would be for Andrew's spine to hold at around 30 degrees.

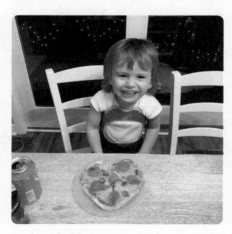

Andrew in his brace.

Despite our disappointment that the casting had stopped working, the transition to bracing brought liberation, Andrew could bathe regularly again and take short breaks for swimming fun. However, this transition also landed during Andrew's fierce two-year-old struggle for independence, which meant that every day we were wrestling with an angry alligator to keep the brace on. That was the only time I ever missed casting, because once a cast is on it stays on! We're thankful this period was short for us and our easygoing Andrew soon returned.

We share our experiences and list of challenges with the hope that others will benefit from what we've learned. While frustrating at times, these specialized circumstances created opportunities for us to observe, listen, understand, and advocate for our son in a very deep way.

On July 2, 2021, 1,166 days, five casts, and two braces following Andrew's scoliosis diagnosis, we received the news we had been praying for: Andrew's curve was maintaining at under 10 degrees. He was cured! We cried, we celebrated, and we seriously considered having a cast-burning bonfire. We were so blessed through casting and bracing. And we could finally celebrate that the years spent worrying about Andrew's future while being so delicately careful with his present were all worth it.

Sarah, mother of 15-year-old Jonathan, with juvenile idiopathic scoliosis (JIS), from Minnesota, US

I never thought much about scoliosis when I was growing up. I remember getting checked for it as a kid, bending over to touch my toes while the doctor looked to make sure my spine was straight. But I never knew anyone with scoliosis until I met my husband. We had been dating only a short while when I noticed that one side of his upper back stuck out more than the other; it was obvious even through his shirt. "Oh, I have scoliosis," he told me.

Never receiving care for it as a child, it was something he had had to live with as an adult. So when our children started having scoliosis checks during their well-child visits, I paid more attention than I maybe otherwise would have.

All our children's reports were good—until Jonathan's at nine years old. The family doctor noted a definite curve and advised that we have it checked out. I knew that scoliosis can run in families, but I was still quite surprised.

We got Jonathan into Gillette Children's right away. After a few visits during which they monitored the curve of Jonathan's spine, we made the decision for him to be fitted for a night brace. It was a tough decision because we knew how hard that would be on him, but we also knew from my husband's experience how important it was to have this corrected in childhood. And Jonathan was about to hit a growth spurt that could worsen the scoliosis, so it was important to start wearing the brace.

The first few nights after Jonathan was fitted for his brace were really hard on him. There is definitely an adjustment period and it is best to ease into wearing it the full night. But after about the first week, he was able to wear it all night without trouble. He had to find the right positions to sleep in, and we went through a few different undershirt styles to find what was most comfortable, but we were all committed to stopping the scoliosis from progressing.

Jon was such a trooper. He would often have to get up at night to change a sweaty undershirt, and we even had to bring the brace with us on vacations (his doctor let him take Christmas and his birthday off!). He loved his scoliosis checks at Gillette because that gave him another sleep free of the brace the night before.

Jon wore the brace for three years. His X-rays had shown us that the brace was working, and that definitely helped him stay the course. The goal of the brace is to stop the scoliosis from progressing, but Jon's X-rays began to show that his curve was actually getting better! We finally got to the point where his curve wasn't even classified as scoliosis anymore, and his doctor agreed to let him do a four-month trial off the brace. Jon, of course, was elated, and even more so when after the trial the X-ray showed no regression.

It has now been 18 months since the brace came off, and we continue to go for checks every 6 months. While Jon is still growing and there's still potential the curve could return, we know that bracing works and will cross that bridge if it comes. We are grateful our family doctor caught the scoliosis early, and so pleased with the team at Gillette who has given our son such wonderful, individualized care.

Jonathan

As a little kid, I remember regular visits to Gillette where we noticed an increasing curve in my back. It was of little concern to me until I was told I had to be fitted with a night brace. I was pretty shaken and quite afraid of how that would affect my life.

The first few nights were hard, but I soon adjusted my routine and the way I slept, and I learned to live with it. The brace was still annoying, but it became just another chore. I absolutely *lived* for my nights off, but wearing the brace definitely didn't destroy my life the way I thought it would.

After a few years, my curve unexpectedly improved, and I was allowed to take a break from the brace! I suppose you never value comfortable sleep until you're deprived of it for three years, but I wouldn't change anything after the way it saved my back. Every cramped night, every sweaty T-shirt, and every boring appointment was 100 percent worth it for such an amazing result. I am now 15 years old and live with no pain and no restrictions. I can play sports, I stand and walk straight, and I no longer have scoliosis!

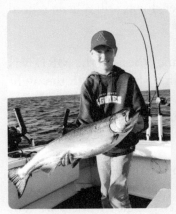 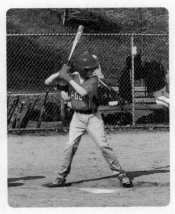

Jonathan fishing and playing baseball after scoliosis brace treatment.

Gracie, a 17-year-old with adolescent idiopathic scoliosis (AIS), from Minnesota, US

On August 8, 2017, age 10 years, my life changed drastically. The trigger for the change happened a couple of days before, when my dad noticed I was standing with one of my shoulders drooping. He told me, "Stand up straight!" and I came back with, "I am!" After that, my dad came over and straightened my shoulders, but they went back to drooping when he let go. That's when we knew something was wrong and immediately booked a chiropractor appointment.

The chiropractor took an X-ray, which revealed my spine was in a complete S-shape. I said it looked exactly like a backward version of the "S" in the logo for Dasani bottled water. We knew then that I needed surgery.

After some research, we landed at Gillette Children's in Minnesota. There is nothing but wonderful things we have to say about our experience there, even for the difficult parts, which included the next step of having an MRI. When I say I hated it, I mean it! I went headfirst into a long scary tube where I had to lie still for 75 minutes. They were truly the worst 75 minutes of my life.

The night before my surgery was Valentine's Day, and we invited all our family and friends to come over and eat cheesecake from the Cheesecake Factory. In a way, it was like a sendoff and good luck for my surgery the next day. I had so much fun with everyone, and it definitely eased most of the anxiety and fear I was feeling. Yet, I was still a little scared for what was to come.

Probably the worst part of this whole experience (besides the MRI) was the dreaded medicine shower. I had to take that shower both the night before and the morning of my surgery to get rid of any lasting bacteria that was on my skin. It was very cold and uncomfortable. We had to also wash my sheets, pajamas, and blankets.

The morning of my surgery I had to wake up really early to be at the hospital in time for my surgery scheduled for 9:30 a.m. The pre-op was so much fun! I got to use some virtual reality goggles while I waited, and my nurse was super funny! They gave me some medicine in my IV that would make me sleepy and told me that I wouldn't remember anything when I woke up.

The next thing I knew was that my surgery was done. I remember after waking up that I needed Chapstick and that they told me to take deep breaths. That night, I wanted to play the Xbox and I played "Are you Smarter than a Fifth Grader?" which I thought was super funny because I was a fifth grader. After that, I fell asleep for the night.

The surgery was very successful. Standing for the first time felt weird but amazing at the same time. I had grown an inch and three-quarters (4.5 cm) after my surgery, and I did feel taller than before. I will never forget that moment.

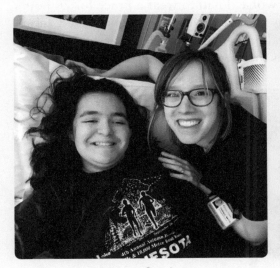 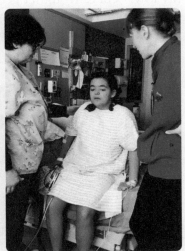

Gracie in the hospital after her surgery.

Before I was allowed to go home, I had to be able to walk upstairs. But that didn't take long; I was in the hospital for only three days after my surgery. My first night at home, my friend Grace came over and we watched movies.

Six days after my surgery, I told my parents that I didn't want to take my pain medication anymore because I didn't like how it made me feel. My parents were afraid that I would be in pain, but we stopped them anyway and, miraculously, I felt great!

A pretty sucky part about the surgery was all my limitations. I had to practice walking and going up and down stairs. (My mom realized that exactly 10 years ago in the same spot she taught me how to walk for the first time.) I couldn't run, jump, twist, bend, ride horses, or lift greater than 10 lb (4.5 kg) for three to four months. I also couldn't swim for four weeks. However, since I had a fast recovery, I was able to return to school sooner than expected. We thought I would be out for up to three weeks, but I made it back in just two and a half weeks. I got back just in time to memorize and learn my part for our spring musical and be in the show. I couldn't participate in recess or P.E., but I got all my makeup homework done.

After my surgery, I got molded for a daytime and a nighttime brace so my lower curve wouldn't get worse. I had to wear a brace for 20 hours a day. My daytime brace was smaller than my nighttime brace. In my nighttime brace, I couldn't walk as it was specifically for sleeping. One thing that was quite funny was that people loved knocking on my brace!

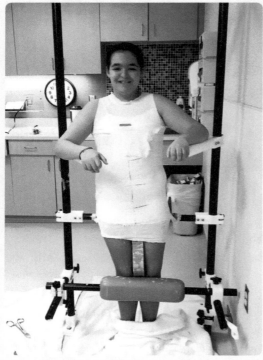

Gracie getting molded for her braces after surgery.

I wore my daytime brace from April 2018 to January 2019, when my spine stopped growing. I continued to have follow-up appointments, which consisted of a meeting with the doctor and having X-rays. I had my last follow-up appointment in summer 2023, and I won't have to have any more of those!

This might sound weird, but my experience was amazing! The nurses were caring, the doctor was skillful, and I hardly had any pain. Everyone made me feel very special, and on the day that I got discharged from the hospital, I didn't want to leave because it was wonderful. It was actually one of the best experiences of my life!

Chapter 7

Further reading and research

Any fool can offer you answers.
It takes a genius to ask the right questions.
Albert Einstein

Further reading

For those who would like further reading on this condition, a list of recommended books, websites, and resources has been collated and will be regularly updated. Access to the list is provided in **Useful web resources.**

Research

Research serves as a cornerstone of evidence-based medicine and drives health care advancement. We discussed the importance of evidence-based medicine (or evidence-based practice) in Chapter 2. It is "the conscientious, explicit, and judicious use of current best evidence in making decisions about the care of individual patients." It combines the best available external clinical evidence from research with the clinical expertise of the professional.[36] Family priorities and preferences are also considered.[132]

Evidence is collected by carrying out scientific studies (research studies), the results of which are published as full-length, peer-reviewed research articles (or papers) in scientific journals. "Peer-reviewed" means that experts with relevant content knowledge have reviewed, challenged, and agreed that the scientific method and study conclusions based on the results are sound.

Scientific studies may also be presented in brief at conferences, and conference proceedings are often published. However, conference proceedings present preliminary results and peer review is minimal. *Therefore, full-length published research articles are the most rigorous and sound evidence.*

The above published research outputs are collectively known as scientific literature or, simply, research.

Research may also be discussed on various social media platforms such as X (formerly Twitter), Facebook, LinkedIn, and Instagram. If you consume information this way, it is always important to go back to the original source (i.e., the full-length research article) to ensure the media's portrayal of the study findings is accurate.

You may have familiarity with searching the scientific literature. If not, search engines such as PubMed (ncbi.nlm.nih.gov/pubmed) and Google Scholar (scholar.google.com) are good places to start. They provide a free abstract (a short summary of the article), which can be very useful. In the past, you generally needed to belong to an academic or medical institution to have access to full-length research articles. Many articles are now available online for free. Google Scholar provides links to many full-length articles, and some community libraries allow you to request full-length articles.

You might have heard the phrase, "Just because someone says it doesn't mean it's true." This is worth remembering in all aspects of life, but it is also relevant to research. While research articles go through a peer review process, you should still read them with a critical eye. Ask yourself, How confident can I be in the results of this research study? Was the sample size big enough to be representative of the larger population? Did the results support the conclusion?

If you aren't a trained scientist, reviewing the quality of the evidence might be more challenging, but you can still make sure the basic methods make sense and the author's conclusions are supported by the data presented. The information below will help you learn about some research study designs and how study design affects how much confidence you can place in a study's conclusions.

Research study design

There are different research study designs, and each has its value. The quality of the evidence, or level of evidence, is graded based on the study design and how well the methods were executed. Research articles sometimes list (often in the abstract) the level of evidence from I to V, with level I being the highest.

The most common research study designs, listed from highest to lowest level of evidence, are:

- Systematic review
- Randomized controlled trial
- Cohort
- Case control
- Cross-sectional
- Case report and case series

Systematic review: A systematic review summarizes the results of several scientific studies on the same topic. They can be qualitative (descriptive) or quantitative (numerical):

- Qualitative: A summary of common themes and findings across studies but without a statistical analysis.
- Quantitative: A statistical analysis carried out that takes a weighted average of the findings across studies to produce one estimate for the effect of a treatment, for example. The quantitative approach is called a "meta-analysis."

The highest level of evidence is a systematic review of randomized controlled trials (described next), although systematic reviews can also include studies that used other types of study designs. Systematic reviews may be published by individual researchers or groups. The Cochrane collaboration is a worldwide association of researchers, health care professionals, patients, and carers that publishes systematic reviews on various topics.

Randomized controlled trial (RCT): An RCT is a study design aimed at identifying cause and effect. The cause is, for example, the treatment, and the effect is the outcome being measured. Strict control of the study method (the "C" in RCT) helps to ensure the treatment of interest is the only factor that could cause the outcome. A treatment group receives the treatment while a nontreatment group (also known as the control group) does not. The participants are randomly assigned (the "R" in RCT) to one of the groups. The random assignment is one of the key strengths of this study design because it takes care of the "unknown unknowns" that may influence the outcome. The treatment effect is found by comparing the outcomes of the treatment and nontreatment groups. RCTs are considered the highest quality study design but are still uncommon in medical literature.

Cohort: A cohort is a group of people who share a common characteristic (e.g., diagnosis, gender). In a cohort study, outcome is measured two or more times. Researchers identify the characteristic of interest and then measure the outcome, looking for associations between the two. A cohort study is a form of longitudinal study ("longitudinal" means that the same outcome is measured on the same participants two or more times over a period of time). You may come across the terms "prospective" and "retrospective" cohort studies.

- In prospective cohort studies, research questions and methods are defined, and a cohort is followed over time, collecting data.
- In retrospective cohort studies, research questions and methods are defined after data has been collected or already exists (e.g., a person's medical record).

Case control: In case control studies, researchers identify the outcome of interest, which defines the groups (e.g., infants with a specific diagnosis and typically developing infants), and then look backward in time at different factors or exposures that might have caused different outcomes. At the beginning of the study, the outcome is known, but the factors or exposures that might have caused that outcome are unknown. This is the opposite of cohort studies. Because the outcome and factors or exposures data already exist, case control studies are always retrospective.

Cross-sectional: Cross-sectional studies take measurements only once from participants. Researchers look for associations between certain factors and exposures, and outcomes.

Case report and case series: A case report (also referred to as a single-subject case study) is an account of a single patient—usually a unique case—and their medical history, status, and outcomes from a treatment, for example. A case series is a group of case reports on patients who were exposed to a similar treatment. These reports are usually retrospective, and data has already been collected by other means (usually as part of routine medical care).

Getting involved in research

There are many opportunities to become involved in research. Together with medical professionals and researchers, people with lived experience can help drive advancement in health care.

a) As a participant

Researchers working in academic and medical settings are always looking for participants for their studies. You might receive an invitation to participate in such a study via an email, letter in the mail, phone call, social media ad, or other method.

Some studies are very easy and may just involve completing one online survey; others may take more time with various measurements being taken on more than one occasion. Just as you are advised to read published research studies with a critical eye, so should you judge new research study opportunities before agreeing to participate. Participating can take time and effort—the expected time commitment will be communicated in the study recruitment material. There is often a small reimbursement offered for time spent in a study.

It's worth noting that you, as the study participant, may not personally benefit from the research study, but the collective population with the condition will likely benefit.

Clinical trials are research studies conducted to evaluate the safety and effectiveness of new medical treatments, including new medications and devices before they can be approved for widespread use. They are often conducted following a randomized controlled trial research study design.

A potential benefit of participating in clinical trials is gaining early access to new medical treatments. Even if you are assigned to the control group (which usually receives standard care), you may have early access to the new treatment once the data collection phase is complete. In addition, standard care is likely to be current best practice.

You can find information about clinical trials through various sources:

- The National Institutes of Health in the US maintains a comprehensive database, ClinicalTrials.gov, where you can learn about clinical trials around the world. You can search this database by specific medical condition, location, or other pertinent criteria to identify relevant clinical trials that may be currently enrolling participants.
- Major academic medical centers, research institutions, and hospitals often conduct clinical trials and can provide information about their ongoing studies.
- Medical professionals may be aware of ongoing clinical trials in their field and can provide guidance to families who are interested in participating.
- Organizations that support particular conditions are another source of information.

Depending on the nature of the treatment in the clinical trial, you may want to, or be required to, consult with your medical professional to help you consider the risks and benefits of participating.

b) As a co-producer

Family engagement in research (FER) plays a crucial role in fostering collaboration and helping improve study design and outcome. When families become involved in research as collaborators on a study rather than simply as participants, researchers gain valuable insights into the lived experiences and perspectives of families. Families participate at every stage of the research process: concept, design, planning, conduct, and reporting of the study findings. These opportunities are still rare but are becoming more common. As an example, a link to the FER program at Gillette Children's is included in **Useful web resources**.

The family engagement in research movement is largely attributed to the similar and earlier patient and public involvement initiative in the UK. Here are some opportunities:

- **CanChild** and the **Kids Brain Health Network** in Canada currently offer The Family Engagement in Research program, a short online training course through McMaster University Continuing Education to train family members and researchers (including coordinators and assistants) in collaborating on research.

- Online training modules are available at **Patient-Oriented Research Curriculum in Child Health (PORCCH)**.
- The **Patient-Centered Outcomes Research Institute (PCORI)** and the **Strategy for Patient-Oriented Research (SPOR)** are two other organizations that encourage family engagement.

USEFUL WEB RESOURCES

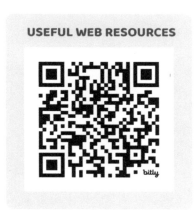

Acknowledgments

It takes a village to raise a child
African proverb

And it takes a village to produce a Healthcare Series. Publication of this series began with an idea, then with five titles, and then more titles. These acknowledgments relate to the entire series.

The formula of deep medical information interspersed with lived experience gives readers an appreciation of the childhood-acquired, often lifelong conditions. We thank the many people who contributed to each title: medical professionals at Gillette Children's who willingly came forward to lead each book; Gillette writers who did the research and writing of each; other Gillette team members who contributed from their different specialties; family authors and vignette writers who shared their personal stories; other families who shared photographs; the Gillette editing team who ensured the content and structure worked for the reader; Olwyn Roche who beautifully illustrated each title; advance readers, both professionals and families, whose feedback was invaluable; and Lina Abdennabi who coordinated Gillette Press operations. Behind every book was also a pit team who converted the finished manuscript into the book you now hold. Ruth Wilson led and looked after copyediting and proofreading. Jazmin Welch created the beautiful design and layout. Audrey McClellan indexed each title.

Smoothly creating each title required great teamwork among our villagers.

Staff at Gillette Children's provided continual support to the project and everyone involved. This included the steering committee, in particular Paula Montgomery, Dr. Micah Niermann, and Barbara Joers.

This Healthcare Series is co-published with Mac Keith Press. From the get-go, the journey with Ann-Marie Halligan and Sally Wilkinson was one of great support and collaboration.

Gillette Children's Healthcare Press

Glossary

TERM	DEFINITION
Adams forward bend test	A clinical exam to identify scoliosis by revealing asymmetry or signs of a rotation and curvature of the spine. The patient bends forward and the provider examines the patient's back from behind.
Adolescent idiopathic scoliosis (AIS)	Idiopathic scoliosis that is diagnosed between the ages of 10 and 18.
Advanced practice provider (APP)	A health care provider who is not a physician but who performs medical activities typically performed by a physician. This includes a physician assistant (PA) and a nurse practitioner (NP), both medical professionals who complete graduate schooling, have greater medical privileges than nurses, and work on the care team.
Alternative treatment	A treatment used in place of conventional medicine.
Alveoli	The air sacs in the lungs that allow for the exchange of oxygen and carbon dioxide.
Anatomical plane	An imaginary division of the body that divides the body into cross-sections; used to show divisions of the body and describe location of structures and direction of movements.
Apical vertebra	The vertebra that is the furthest away from the center of the body for a given scoliosis curve.
Axial plane	An anatomical plane that separates the upper and lower halves of the body. As the observer looking at the axial plane of the body, you are above a standing person, looking down at the top of their head. Also called the transverse plane.
Cardiopulmonary	Referring to the heart (cardio) and lungs (pulmonary).

Cobb angle	The most commonly used measurement for quantifying the size of a spinal curve, also called the curve magnitude.
Complementary treatment	A treatment used together with conventional medicine.
Computerized tomography (CT) scan	A noninvasive imaging technology that uses a series of X-rays to create detailed images of the bones and soft tissues.
Congenital	Referring to a condition that is present from birth.
Congenital scoliosis	Scoliosis that develops due to errors in vertebral development.
Connective tissue	Tissue that connects, supports, binds, or separates other tissues or organs; examples include bone, blood vessels, cartilage, ligaments, and tendons.
Coronal plane	An anatomical plane that separates the front and back of the body. As the observer looking at the coronal plane of the body, you are looking at a person who is facing you straight on or away from you. Also called the frontal plane.
Disc degeneration	A breakdown and thinning of the intervertebral discs.
Early-onset scoliosis (EOS)	Scoliosis that is diagnosed prior to 10 years of age.
Evidence-based medicine	The conscientious, explicit, and judicious use of current best evidence in making decisions about the care of individual patients.
Facet joints	The area along the back of the spine where two vertebrae meet. Like most joints in the body, facet joints provide movement and flexibility to the spine.
First-degree family member	A parent, child, or full sibling.
Growth-friendly treatment	A type of spine surgery where the scoliosis curve is straightened, and expandable metal rods are inserted and lengthened over time for continued curve correction.
Growth plate	Area of active, new bone growth that is made of cartilage and turns to solid bone when growing is done.

Halo gravity traction	A multistage treatment for severe scoliosis to stretch and straighten the spine and soft tissues (skin, muscle, ligaments) prior to scoliosis surgery.
Health care transition	The planned process and skill-building to empower adolescents and their families to navigate an adult model of health care.
Health-related quality of life (HRQOL)	An individual's or a group's perceived physical and mental health over time.
Hyperkyphosis	Excessive rounding of the spine, typically in the thoracic region.
Hyperlordosis	Excessive arching of the spine, typically in the lumbar region; can also develop in the cervical region.
Hypokyphosis	A loss of kyphosis and the presentation of an abnormally straight or flat spine, typically in the thoracic region.
Hypolordosis	A loss of lordosis and the presentation of an abnormally straight or flat spine, typically in the lumbar region.
Idiopathic	Relating to a disease of unknown cause.
Idiopathic scoliosis	Scoliosis that develops from an unknown cause.
Infantile idiopathic scoliosis (IIS)	Idiopathic scoliosis that is diagnosed between birth and age three.
Intervertebral disc	A cartilage structure that sits between vertebral bodies and offers shock absorption during movement, as well as increased flexibility.
Intervertebral foramen	The opening between each vertebra that allows nerves to branch off the spinal cord and travel to other parts of the body.
Juvenile idiopathic scoliosis (JIS)	Idiopathic scoliosis that is diagnosed between four and nine years of age.
Kyphosis	An outward curvature of the spine, rounding away from the center of the body.
Long-term surgical complication	Problems that may occur after the individual has been discharged from the hospital and may develop over the course of months or even years following surgery.

Lordosis	An inward curvature of the spine, arching toward the center of the body.
Lower instrumented vertebra	The lowest vertebra (closest to the tailbone) that is instrumented (has screws or hooks) in it.
Magnetically controlled growing rods (MCGRs)	Adjustable metal rods that can be lengthened via a magnetic external remote control and are attached to the spine with screws or hooks.
Magnetic resonance imaging (MRI)	A noninvasive imaging technology that produces detailed three-dimensional anatomical images without the use of radiation; allows for detailed imaging of soft-tissue internal structures in the body.
Metallosis	The buildup of metal debris in the soft tissues of the body.
Natural history study	A research study that collects information about the progression of a disease over time without any intervention.
Neural axis abnormality	A condition characterized by atypical structures within the central nervous system (brain and/or spinal cord).
Neurologic injury	Injury to the spinal cord or nerves resulting in temporary or permanent loss of function or sensation.
Neuromuscular condition	A condition involving the nervous system and/or muscles.
Neuromuscular scoliosis	Scoliosis that develops secondary to a neuromuscular condition.
Nighttime hypercorrective TLSO	A spinal orthosis (brace) prescribed to be worn only while lying down, typically when an individual is sleeping.
Orthotist	A health care professional who designs and fits orthoses (braces).
Osteoarthritis	Cartilage breakdown in the facet joints of the spine.
Osteopenia	Bone density that is not typical but not as low as osteoporosis.
Osteoporosis	A loss in bone density that is significantly lower than typical for a person's age.

Pedicle	A bony bridge located on the left and right side of each vertebra, connecting the front of the vertebra to the back of the vertebra.
Physical therapy scoliosis-specific exercises (PSSE)	A type of physical therapy available to individuals with scoliosis that aims to help the individual control their posture through stretching, strengthening, posture corrections, breathing exercises, and education.
Pleural effusion	Excess collection of fluid surrounding the lungs.
Pneumothorax	Partial or complete lung collapse.
Proximal humerus ossification system (PHOS)	A skeletal maturity scoring system that observes the growth plate in the upper arm bone.
Proximal junctional kyphosis (PJK)	Hyperkyphosis that develops above the upper instrumented vertebra that can weaken the connection between the screws and bone, causing the screws to pull out of the bone and/or for the instrumentation to be prominent (visible through the skin).
Pseudoarthrosis	The failure of fusion; the failure of bones to unite properly.
Psychosocial	Referring to both psychological and social factors.
Rib phase	A description of the proximity of the rib to the apical vertebra on an X-ray; in phase 1, there is a gap between the rib and the vertebra, and in phase 2, the rib appears to overlap the vertebra.
Rib vertebral angle difference (RVAD)	A measurement of the difference in angles between the two ribs attached to the apical vertebra.
Risk factor	Any attribute, characteristic, or exposure of an individual that increases the likelihood of developing a disease or injury.
Risser sign	A skeletal maturity scoring system that observes the growth plate that forms across the top of each side of the pelvis.
Sagittal plane	An anatomical plane that separates the left and right sides of the body. As the observer looking at the sagittal plane of the body, you are looking at the side view of a person. Also called the lateral plane.

Sanders stage	A skeletal maturity scoring system that observes the growth plates in the bones of the hand and wrist.
Scoliometer	A specifically designed level used to measure the degree of vertebral rotation in the spine.
Scoliosis	A condition in which there is an atypical three-dimensional curvature and rotation of the spine of at least 10 degrees.
Scoliosis Research Society Instrument 22-R (SRS-22r)	A scoliosis-specific questionnaire on pain, function, self-image, mental health, and satisfaction with care.
Sign	An indication of a disease or condition; what can be seen by observing the individual.
Spinal canal	The hole through each of the vertebrae; where the spinal cord passes through.
Spinal fusion	A type of spine surgery where two or more vertebrae are fused (joined together) to stop curve progression and improve the angle of the curve (decrease the Cobb angle).
Spine	The skeletal, or bony, structure that surrounds the spinal cord.
Surgical risk	Complications that may occur in or shortly after surgery while the individual is still in the hospital; also called an in-hospital complication.
Symptom	What an individual describes as experiencing due to a disease or condition.
Syndrome	A group of symptoms that consistently occur together.
Syndromic scoliosis	Scoliosis that develops secondary to a syndrome.
Thoracic height	The length of the thoracic region of the spine.
Thoracic insufficiency syndrome	The inability of the thorax (spine, ribs, and sternum) to allow for normal breathing or lung growth.
Thoraco-lumbo-sacral orthosis (TLSO)	A spinal brace made of molded, rigid plastic that extends from the armpits to the pelvis, not limiting hip motion; used to stop scoliosis curve progression.

Traditional growing rods	Metal rods that are manually lengthened during surgery under general anesthesia.
Triradiate cartilage	A skeletal maturity scoring system that observes the growth plates in the hip joint.
Upper instrumented vertebra	The highest vertebra (closest to the head) that is instrumented (has screws or hooks) in it.
Vertebrae	Individual bones of the spine with a hole in the middle for the spinal cord to pass through.
Vertebral body	The column-shaped part of the vertebra that bears the majority of the load or body weight.
Vertebral body tethering (VBT)	A type of spine surgery where screws are inserted and a rope (tether), that is under tension, is attached to the convex side of the scoliosis curve (the outside of the curve).

References

1. World Health Organization (2001) *International classification of functioning, disability and health (ICF)*. [online] Available at: <https://www.who.int/standards/classifications/international-classification-of-functioning-disability-and-health> [Accessed February 22 2024].

2. Illes T, Tunyogi-Csapo M, Somoskeoy S (2011) Breakthrough in three-dimensional scoliosis diagnosis: Significance of horizontal plane view and vertebra vectors. *Eur Spine J*, 20, 135-43.

3. Yaszay B, Newton O (2021) Idiopathic scoliosis. In: Weinstein S, Flynn J, Crawford H, editors, *Lovell and Winter's pediatric orthopaedics* 8th ed. Philadelphia: Wolters Kluwer, pp 659-720.

4. American Association of Neurological Surgeons (2023) *Scoliosis*. [online] Available at: <https://www.aans.org/Patients/Neurosurgical-Conditions-and-Treatments/Scoliosis> [Accessed April 23 2024].

5. Roussouly P, Nnadi C (2010) Sagittal plane deformity: An overview of interpretation and management. *Eur Spine J*, 19, 1824-36.

6. Breeland G, Sinkler MA, Menezes RG (2023) *Embryology, bone ossification*. [e-book] Treasure Island (FL), StatPearls Publishing. Available at: National Library of Medicine <www.ncbi.nlm.nih.gov/books/NBK539718/>.

7. Scoliosis Research Society (2023a) *Diagnosis & screening of scoliosis*. [online] Available at: <https://www.srs.org/Patients/Diagnosis-And-Treatment/Diagnosing-Scoliosis> [Accessed April 22 2024].

8. Gillette Children's (2023a) *Scoliosis (idiopathic, neuromuscular and congenital)*. [online] Available at: <https://www.gillettechildrens.org/conditions-care/scoliosis-idiopathic-neuromuscular-and-congenital/what-is-scoliosis> [Accessed June 15 2023].

9. Thuaimer A, Knipe H, Elfeky M (2023) Cobb angle. *Radiopaedia*. [online] Available at: <https://radiopaedia.org/articles/23612> [Accessed April 24 2024].

10. Williams BA, McClung A, Blakemore LC, et al. (2020) MRI utilization and rates of abnormal pretreatment MRI findings in early-onset scoliosis: Review of a global cohort. *Spine Deform*, 8, 1099-1107.

11. Simony A, Carreon LY, Hojmark K, Kyvik KO, Andersen M (2016) Concordance rates of adolescent idiopathic scoliosis in a Danish twin population. *Spine*, 41, 1503-1507.

12. Konieczny MR, Senyurt H, Krauspe R (2013) Epidemiology of adolescent idiopathic scoliosis. *J Child Orthop*, 7, 3-9.

13. Centers for Disease Control and Prevention (2015) *Epidemiology glossary*. [online] Available at: <https://www.cdc.gov/reproductivehealth/data_stats/glossary.html> [Accessed January 19 2024].

14. Thorsness RJ, Faust JR, Behrend CJ, Sanders JO (2015) Nonsurgical management of early-onset scoliosis. *J Am Acad Orthop Surg,* 23, 519-28.

15. Mehta MH (1972) The rib-vertebra angle in the early diagnosis between resolving and progressive infantile scoliosis. *J Bone Joint Surg Br,* 54, 230-43.

16. Robinson CM, McMaster MJ (1996) Juvenile idiopathic scoliosis. Curve patterns and prognosis in one hundred and nine patients. *J Bone Joint Surg Am,* 78, 1140-8.

17. Lenke LG, Dobbs MB (2007) Management of juvenile idiopathic scoliosis. *J Bone Joint Surg Am,* 89, 55-63.

18. Agabegi SS, Kazemi N, Sturm PF, Mehlman CT (2015) Natural history of adolescent idiopathic scoliosis in skeletally mature patients: A critical review. *J Am Acad Orthop Surg,* 23, 714-23.

19. Li S, Yang J, Li Y, et al. (2013) Right ventricular function impaired in children and adolescents with severe idiopathic scoliosis. *Scoliosis,* 8, 1-7.

20. Campbell RM, Jr., Smith MD, Mayes TC, et al. (2003) The characteristics of thoracic insufficiency syndrome associated with fused ribs and congenital scoliosis. *J Bone Joint Surg Am,* 85, 399-408.

21. Flynn JM, Hasler CC, Vitale MG (2021) Early-onset spine deformities. In: Weinstein S, Flynn JM, editors, *Lovell and Winter's pediatric orthopaedics.* 8th ed. Philadelphia: Wolters Kluwer, pp 721-750.

22. Rehman S, Bacha D (2023) *Embryology, pulmonary.* [e-book] Treasure Island (FL), StatPearls. Available at: National Library of Medicine <https://www.ncbi.nlm.nih.gov/books/NBK544372/> [Accessed May 22 2024].

23. Pehrsson K, Larsson S, Oden A, Nachemson A (1992) Long-term follow-up of patients with untreated scoliosis. A study of mortality, causes of death, and symptoms. *Spine,* 17, 1091-6.

24. Weinstein SL, Dolan LA, Spratt KF, et al. (2003) Health and function of patients with untreated idiopathic scoliosis: A 50-year natural history study. *JAMA,* 289, 559-67.

25. Makhni MC, Shillingford JN, Laratta JL, Hyun SJ, Kim YJ (2018) Restoration of sagittal balance in spinal deformity surgery. *J Korean Neurosurg Soc,* 61, 167-179.

26. Belli G, Toselli S, Latessa PM, Mauro M (2022) Evaluation of self-perceived body image in adolescents with mild idiopathic scoliosis. *Eur J Investig Health Psychol Educ,* 12, 319-333.

27. Zhang J, He D, Gao J, et al. (2011) Changes in life satisfaction and self-esteem in patients with adolescent idiopathic scoliosis with and without surgical intervention. *Spine,* 36, 741-5.

28. Carrasco MIB, Ruiz MCS (2016) Idiopathic adolescent scoliosis: Living with a physical deformity. *Texto & Contexto - Enfermagem,* 25, 1-9.

29. Cheng JC, Castelein RM, Chu WC, et al. (2015) Adolescent idiopathic scoliosis. *Nature Reviews Disease Primers,* 1, 1-21.

30. Sanders JO, Khoury JG, Kishan S, et al. (2008) Predicting scoliosis progression from skeletal maturity: A simplified classification during adolescence. *J Bone Joint Surg Am,* 90, 540-53.

31. Dimeglio A, Canavese F (2012) Progression or not progression? How to deal with adolescent idiopathic scoliosis during puberty. *J Child Orthop*, 7, 43-9.

32. Weinstein SL, Dolan LA, Wright JG, Dobbs MB (2013) Effects of bracing in adolescents with idiopathic scoliosis. *N Engl J Med*, 369, 1512-21.

33. Katz DE, Herring JA, Browne RH, Kelly DM, Birch JG (2010) Brace wear control of curve progression in adolescent idiopathic scoliosis. *J Bone Joint Surg Am*, 92, 1343-52.

34. Smith K, Benish B, Nelson E, et al. (2024) The effect of thoraco-lumbo-sacral orthosis wear time and clinical risk factors on curve progression for individuals with adolescent idiopathic scoliosis. [online] Available at: <https://www.science direct.com/science/article/pii/S152994302400891X?dgcid=author> [Accessed August 13 2024].

35. Karol LA, Virostek D, Felton K, Jo C, Butler L (2016) The effect of the Risser stage on bracing outcome in adolescent idiopathic scoliosis. *J Bone Joint Surg Am*, 98, 1253-9.

36. Sackett DL, Rosenberg WM, Gray JA, Haynes RB, Richardson WS (1996) Evidence-based medicine: What it is and what it isn't. *BMJ*, 312, 71-2.

37. Siminoff LA (2013) Incorporating patient and family preferences into evidence-based medicine. *BMC Med Inform Decis Mak*, 13, 1-7.

38. Agency for Healthcare Research and Quality (2020) *The SHARE approach: A model for shared decisionmaking - fact sheet.* [online] Available at: <https://www.ahrq.gov/health-literacy/professional-training/shared-decision/tools/factsheet.html> [Accessed January 19 2024].

39. Yang Y, Han X, Chen Z, et al. (2023) Bone mineral density in children and young adults with idiopathic scoliosis: A systematic review and meta-analysis. *Eur Spine J*, 32, 149-166.

40. Lam Tp, Hon Kei Yip B, Chi Wai Man G, et al. (2017). Effective therapeutic control of curve progression using calcium and vitamin D supplementation for adolescent idiopathic scoliosis – a randomized double-blinded placebo-controlled trial. [online] Available at: <https://www.bone-abstracts.org/ba/0006/ba0006oc8> [Accessed April 23 2024].

41. Scoliosis Research Society (2023b) *Treating scoliosis.* [online] Available at: <https://www.srs.org/Patients/Diagnosis-And-Treatment/Bracing> [Accessed April 23 2024].

42. Gillette Children's (2023b) *Casting and bracing.* [online] Available at: <https://www.gillettechildrens.org/conditions-care/spinal-bracing-and-casting> [Accessed April 23 2024].

43. Buyuk AF, Truong WH, Morgan SJ, et al. (2022) Is nighttime bracing effective in the treatment of adolescent idiopathic scoliosis? A meta-analysis and systematic review based on scoliosis research society guidelines. *Spine Deform*, 10, 247-256.

44. Cheung PWH, Cheung JPY (2021) Sanders stage 7b: Using the appearance of the ulnar physis improves decision-making for brace weaning in patients with adolescent idiopathic scoliosis. *Bone Joint J*, 103-b, 141-147.

45. Richards BS, Bernstein RM, D'Amato CR, Thompson GH (2005) Standardization of criteria for adolescent idiopathic scoliosis brace studies: SRS committee on bracing and nonoperative management. *Spine*, 30, 2068-2075.

46. Hawary RE, Zaaroor-Regev D, Floman Y, et al. (2019) Brace treatment in adolescent idiopathic scoliosis: Risk factors for failure – a literature review. *Spine J*, 19, 1917-1925.

47. Warren J, Hey L, Mazzoleni A (2022) Biomechanical analysis of the impact of increasing levels of body mass index on the ability of a bracing orthosis to alter the asymmetric compressive growth plate loading in a scoliotic spine. *Biomedical Engineering Advances*, 4, 1-7.

48. Dolan LA, Weinstein SL, Abel MF, et al. (2019) Bracing in adolescent idiopathic scoliosis trial (BrAIST): Development and validation of a prognostic model in untreated adolescent idiopathic scoliosis using the simplified skeletal maturity system. *Spine Deform*, 7, 890-898.

49. Wang H, Tetteroo D, Arts JJC, Markopoulos P, Ito K (2021) Quality of life of adolescent idiopathic scoliosis patients under brace treatment: A brief communication of literature review. *Qual Life Res*, 30, 703-711.

50. Rahimi S, Kiaghadi A, Fallahian N (2020) Effective factors on brace compliance in idiopathic scoliosis: A literature review. *Disabil Rehabil Assist Technol*, 15, 917-923.

51. Benish BM, Smith KJ, Schwartz MH (2012) Validation of a miniature thermochron for monitoring thoracolumbosacral orthosis wear time. *Spine*, 37, 309-15.

52. Karol LA, Virostek D, Felton K, Wheeler L (2016) Effect of compliance counseling on brace use and success in patients with adolescent idiopathic scoliosis. *J Bone Joint Surg Am*, 98, 9-14.

53. Law D, Cheung MC, Yip J, Yick KL, Wong C (2017) Scoliosis brace design: Influence of visual aesthetics on user acceptance and compliance. *Ergonomics*, 60, 876-886.

54. Schwieger T, Campo S, Steuber KR, Weinstein SL, Ashida S (2016) An exploration of information exchange by adolescents and parents participating in adolescent idiopathic scoliosis online support groups. *Scoliosis and Spinal Disorders*, 11, 1-7.

55. Laquièvre A, Dolet N, Moisson L, et al. (2020) Compliance with night-time overcorrection bracing in adolescent idiopathic scoliosis: Result from a cohort follow-up. *Med Eng Phys*, 77, 137-141.

56. Mehta MH (2005) Growth as a corrective force in the early treatment of progressive infantile scoliosis. *J Bone Joint Surg Br*, 87, 1237-47.

57. Welborn M, Sanders J, Astous J (2021) The evolution of EDF casting: Current concept review. *Journal of the Pediatric Orthopaedic Society of North America*, 3, 1-8.

58. Sanders JO, D'astous J, Fitzgerald M, et al. (2009) Derotational casting for progressive infantile scoliosis. *J Pediatr Orthop*, 29, 581-7.

59. Fedorak GT, Stasikelis PJ, Carpenter AM, Nielson AN, D'astous JL (2019) Optimization of casting in early-onset scoliosis. *J Pediatr Orthop*, 39, 303-307.

60. Welborn MC, D'Astous J, Bratton S, Heflin J (2018) Infantile idiopathic scoliosis: Factors affecting EDF casting success. *Spine Deform*, 6, 614-620.

61. Fedorak GT, MacWilliams BA, Stasikelis P, et al. (2022) Age-stratified outcomes of Mehta casting in idiopathic early-onset scoliosis: A multicenter review. *J Bone Joint Surg Am*, 104, 1977-1983.

62. Gomez JA, Grzywna A, Miller PE, et al. (2017) Initial cast correction as a predictor of treatment outcome success for infantile idiopathic scoliosis. *J Pediatr Orthop*, 37, 625-630.

63. Alassaf N, Tabard-Fougère A, Dayer R (2020) Casting in infantile idiopathic scoliosis as a temporising measure: A systematic review and meta-analysis. *SAGE Open Med*, 8, 1-7.

64. Lavalva S, Adams A, Macalpine E, et al. (2020) Serial casting in neuromuscular and syndromic early-onset scoliosis (EOS) can delay surgery over 2 years. *J Pediatr Orthop*, 40, 772-779.

65. Demirkiran HG, Bekmez S, Celilov R, et al. (2015) Serial derotational casting in congenital scoliosis as a time-buying strategy. *J Pediatr Orthop*, 35, 43-9.

66. Matsumoto H, Auran E, Fields MW, et al. (2020) Serial casting for early onset scoliosis and its effects on health-related quality of life during and after discontinuation of treatment. *Spine Deformity*, 8, 1361-1367.

67. Henstenburg J, Heard J, Sturm P, et al. (2023) Does transitioning to a brace improve HRQOL after casting for early onset scoliosis? *Journal of Pediatric Orthopaedics*, 43, 151-155.

68. Centers for Disease Control and Prevention (2021) *Health-related quality of life (HRQOL)*. [online] Available at: <https://archive.cdc.gov/#/details?url=https://www.cdc.gov/hrqol/index.htm> [Accessed April 22 2024].

69. U.S. Food and Drug Administration (2016) *FDA drug safety communication: FDA review results in new warnings about using general anesthetics and sedation drugs in young children and pregnant women.* [online] Available at: <https://www.fda.gov/drugs/drug-safety-and-availability/fda-drug-safety-communication-fda-review-results-new-warnings-about-using-general-anesthetics-and> [Accessed April 23 2024].

70. Xiao A, Feng Y, Yu S, et al. (2022) General anesthesia in children and long-term neurodevelopmental deficits: A systematic review. *Front Mol Neurosci*, 15, 1-23.

71. LaValva S, MacAlpine EM, Kawakami N, et al. (2020) Awake serial body casting for the management of infantile idiopathic scoliosis: Is general anesthesia necessary? *Spine Deformity*, 8, 1109-1115.

72. Fedorak GT, Dreksler H, MacWilliams BA, D'Astous JL (2020) What is the cost of a "cast holiday" in treating children with early onset scoliosis (EOS) with elongation derotation flexion (EDF, "Mehta") casting? *J Pediatr Orthop*, 40, 396-400.

73. World Confederation for Physical Therapy (2023) *What is physiotherapy?* [online] Available at: <https://world.physio/resources/what-is-physiotherapy> [Accessed February 22 2024].

74. Scoliosis Research Society (2023c) *Scoliosis*. [online] Available at: <https://www.srs.org/Patients/Conditions/Scoliosis> [Accessed April 23 2024].

75. Negrini S, Donzelli S, Aulisa AG, et al. (2018) 2016 SOSORT guidelines: Orthopaedic and rehabilitation treatment of idiopathic scoliosis during growth. *Scoliosis and Spinal Disorders*, 13, 1-48.

76. Edemekong PF, Bomgaars Dl, Sukumaran S, Schoo C (2023) *Activities of daily living.* [online] Available at: <https://www.ncbi.nlm.nih.gov/books/NBK470404/> [Accessed April 20 2024].

77. Weiss H-R (2011) The method of Katharina Schroth - History, principles and current development. *Scoliosis*, 6, 1-21.

78. Gillette Children's (2023c) *Physical therapy for scoliosis.* [online] Available at: <https://www.gillettechildrens.org/conditions-care/physical-therapy-for-scoliosis> [Accessed April 23 2024].

79. Seleviciene V, Cesnaviciute A, Strukcinskiene B, et al. (2022) Physiotherapeutic scoliosis-specific exercise methodologies used for conservative treatment of adolescent idiopathic scoliosis, and their effectiveness: An extended literature review of current research and practice. *Int J Environ Res Public Health*, 19, 1-19.

80. Tolo VT, Herring JA (2020) Scoliosis-specific exercises: A state of the art review. *Spine Deform*, 8, 149-155.

81. Gao A, Li JY, Shao R, et al. (2021) Schroth exercises improve health-related quality of life and radiographic parameters in adolescent idiopathic scoliosis patients. *Chin Med J (Engl)*, 134, 2589-2596.

82. Schreiber S, Parent EC, Moez EK, et al. (2015) The effect of Schroth exercises added to the standard of care on the quality of life and muscle endurance in adolescents with idiopathic scoliosis – an assessor and statistician blinded randomized controlled trial: "SOSORT 2015 award winner." *Scoliosis*, 10, 1-12.

83. National Center for Complementary and Integrative Health (2023) *Complementary, alternative, or integrative health: What's in a name?* [online] Available at: <https://www.nccih.nih.gov/health/complementary-alternative-or -integrative-health-whats-in-a-name> [Accessed April 23 2024].

84. McAviney J (2013) Chiropractic treatment of scoliosis; a systematic review of the scientific literature. *Scoliosis*, 8, 1-1.

85. Woggon AJ, Woggon DA (2015) Patient-reported side effects immediately after chiropractic scoliosis treatment: A cross-sectional survey utilizing a practice-based research network. *Scoliosis*, 10, 1-6.

86. Choi Seong-Kyeong, Jo Hyo-Rim, Moon Jeong-Hyun, et al. (2022) Effectiveness of acupuncture for scoliosis: A systematic review. *Journal of Acupuncture Research*, 39, 17-28.

87. Johnston CE, Karol LA, Thornberg D, Jo C, Eamara P (2021) The 18-cm thoracic-height threshold and pulmonary function in non-neuromuscular early-onset scoliosis: A reassessment. *JB JS Open Access*, 6, 1-9.

88. Lavelle W, Kurra S, Hu X, Lieberman I (2020) Clinical outcomes of idiopathic scoliosis surgery: Is there a difference between young adult patients and adolescent patients? *Cureus*, 12, 1-9.

89. American Society of Anesthesiologists (2023) *Anesthesia risks.* [online] Available at: <https://www.asahq.org/madeforthismoment/anesthesia-101/types-of-anesthesia/ anesthesia-risks/> [Accessed April 23 2024].

90. De La Garza Ramos R, Goodwin CR, Abu-Bonsrah N, et al. (2016) Patient and operative factors associated with complications following adolescent idiopathic scoliosis surgery: An analysis of 36,335 patients from the nationwide inpatient sample. *J Neurosurg Pediatr*, 25, 730-736.

91. Lee J, Park YS (2016) Proximal junctional kyphosis: Diagnosis, pathogenesis, and treatment. *Asian Spine J*, 10, 593-600.

92. Hariharan AR, Shah SA, Petfield J, et al. (2022) Complications following surgical treatment of adolescent idiopathic scoliosis: A 10-year prospective follow-up study. *Spine Deform*, 10, 1097-1105.

93. Shin M, Arguelles GR, Cahill PJ, et al. (2021) Complications, reoperations, and mid-term outcomes following anterior vertebral body tethering versus posterior spinal fusion: A meta-analysis. *JB JS Open Access*, 6, 1-9.

94. Bess S, Akbarnia BA, Thompson GH, et al. (2010) Complications of growing-rod treatment for early-onset scoliosis: Analysis of one hundred and forty patients. *J Bone Joint Surg Am*, 92, 2533-43.

95. Thakar C, Kieser DC, Mardare M, et al. (2018) Systematic review of the complications associated with magnetically controlled growing rods for the treatment of early onset scoliosis. *Eur Spine J*, 27, 2062-2071.

96. Gov.Uk (2024) *Targeted communication: CE mark suspended for all MAGEC systems manufactured by Nuvasive Specialized Orthopedics, Inc. (dsi/2021/007).* [online] Available at: <https://www.gov.uk/drug-device-alerts/targeted-communication-ce-mark-suspended-for-all-magec-systems-manufactured-by-nuvasive-specialized-orthopedics-inc> [Accessed April 23 2024].

97. Flynn JM, Tomlinson LA, Pawelek J, et al. (2013) Growing-rod graduates: Lessons learned from ninety-nine patients who completed lengthening. *J Bone Joint Surg Am*, 95, 1745-50.

98. Vatkar A, Najjar E, Patel M, Quraishi NA (2023) Vertebral body tethering in adolescent idiopathic scoliosis with more than 2 years of follow-up - systematic review and meta-analysis. *Eur Spine J*, 32, 3047-3057.

99. U.S. Food and Drug Administration (2023a) *Humanitarian device exemption (HDE).* [online] Available at: <https://www.accessdata.fda.gov/scripts/cdrh/cfdocs/cfhde/hde.cfm?id=H190005> [Accessed April 23 2024].

100. U.S. Food and Drug Administration (2023b) *Humanitarian use device (HUD) designation program.* [online] Available at: <https://www.fda.gov/industry/medical-products-rare-diseases-and-conditions/humanitarian-use-device-hud-designation-program> [Accessed 2024 April 23].

101. Newton PO (2020) Spinal growth tethering: Indications and limits. *Ann Transl Med*, 8, 1-7.

102. Hammad AM, Balsano M, Ahmad AA (2023) Vertebral body tethering: An alternative to posterior spinal fusion in idiopathic scoliosis? *Front Pediatr*, 1, 1-11.

103. Roser MJ, Askin GN, Labrom RD, et al. (2023) Vertebral body tethering for idiopathic scoliosis: A systematic review and meta-analysis. *Spine Deform*, 11, 1297-1307.

104. Jackson TJ, Sullivan MH, Larson AN, Milbrandt TA, Sebastian AS (2023) Controversies in spine surgery: Is vertebral body tethering superior to selective thoracic fusion for adolescent idiopathic scoliosis? *Clinical Spine Surgery*, 36, 291-294.

105. Wong DLL, Mong PT, Ng CY, et al. (2023) Can anterior vertebral body tethering provide superior range of motion outcomes compared to posterior spinal fusion in adolescent idiopathic scoliosis? A systematic review. *Eur Spine J*, 32, 3058-3071.

106. Pahys JM, Samdani AF, Hwang SW, et al., (2022) Trunk range of motion and patient outcomes after anterior vertebral body tethering versus posterior spinal fusion: Comparison using computerized 3D motion capture technology. *J Bone Joint Surg Am,* 104, 1563-1572.

107. Polly DW, Larson AN, Samdani AF, et al. (2021) Cost-utility analysis of anterior vertebral body tethering versus spinal fusion in idiopathic scoliosis from a US integrated healthcare delivery system perspective. *Clinicoecon Outcomes Res,* 13, 175-190.

108. Centers for Disease Control and Prevention (2017) *Characteristics of initial prescription episodes and likelihood of long-term opioid use — United States, 2006-2015.* [online] Available at: <https://www.cdc.gov/mmwr/volumes/66/wr/mm6610a1.htm> [Accessed April 23 2024].

109. Wheatley BM, Nappo KE, Christensen DL, et al., (2019) Effect of NSAIDS on bone healing rates: A meta-analysis. *J Am Acad Orthop Surg,* 27, 330-336.

110. Gomez JA, Lee JK, Kim PD, Roye DP, Vitale MG (2011) "Growth friendly" spine surgery: Management options for the young child with scoliosis. *J Am Acad Orthop Surg,* 19, 722-7.

111. Yang Z, Liu Y, Qi L, et al. (2021) Does preoperative halo-gravity traction reduce the degree of deformity and improve pulmonary function in severe scoliosis patients with pulmonary insufficiency? A systematic review and meta-analysis. *Front Med (Lausanne),* 8, 1-8.

112. Popescu MB, Ulici A, Carp M, Haram O, Ionescu NS (2022) The use and complications of halo gravity traction in children with scoliosis. *Children,* 9, 1-11.

113. Iyer S, Duah HO, Wulff I, et al. (2019) The use of halo gravity traction in the treatment of severe early onset spinal deformity. *Spine,* 44, 841-845.

114. Bogunovic L, Lenke LG, Bridwell KH, Luhmann SJ (2013) Preoperative halo-gravity traction for severe pediatric spinal deformity: Complications, radiographic correction and changes in pulmonary function. *Spine Deform,* 1, 33-39.

115. Rocos B, Reda L, Lebel D, Dodds M, Zeller R (2021) The use of halo gravity traction in severe, stiff scoliosis. *J Pediatr Orthop,* 41, 338-343.

116. Hwang CJ, Kim DG, Lee CS, et al. (2020) Preoperative halo traction for severe scoliosis. *Spine,* 45, 1158-1165.

117. Benoist M (2003) Natural history of the aging spine. *Eur Spine J,* 12, 86-9.

118. Danielsson AJ, Nachemson AL (2001) Radiologic findings and curve progression 22 years after treatment for adolescent idiopathic scoliosis: Comparison of brace and surgical treatment with matching control group of straight individuals. *Spine,* 26, 516-25.

119. Bisson GD, Lama P, Abduljabbar F, et al. (2018) Facet joint degeneration in adolescent idiopathic scoliosis. *JOR Spine,* 1, 1-11.

120. National Institute on Aging (2023) *Osteoporosis.* [online] Available at: <https://www.nia.nih.gov/health/osteoporosis/osteoporosis> [Accessed April 23 2024].

121. Nicholson T, Scott A, Newton Ede M, Jones SW (2021) Do e-cigarettes and vaping have a lower risk of osteoporosis, nonunion, and infection than tobacco smoking? *Bone Joint Res,* 10, 188-191.

122. Asher MA, Lai SM, Glattes RC, et al. (2006) Refinement of the SRS-22 health-related quality of life questionnaire function domain. *Spine,* 31, 593-7.

123. Diarbakerli E, Grauers A, Danielsson A, Gerdhem P (2017) Adults with idiopathic scoliosis diagnosed at youth experience similar physical activity and fracture rate as controls. *Spine,* 42, 404-410.
124. Danielsson AJ, Wiklund I, Pehrsson K, Nachemson AL (2001) Health-related quality of life in patients with adolescent idiopathic scoliosis: A matched follow-up at least 20 years after treatment with brace or surgery. *Eur Spine J,* 10, 278-88.
125. Andersen MO, Christensen SB, Thomsen K (2006) Outcome at 10 years after treatment for adolescent idiopathic scoliosis. *Spine,* 31, 350-4.
126. Pehrsson K, Danielsson A, Nachemson A (2001) Pulmonary function in adolescent idiopathic scoliosis: A 25 year follow up after surgery or start of brace treatment. *Thorax,* 56, 388-93.
127. Topalis C, Grauers A, Diarbakerli E, Danielsson A, Gerdhem P (2017) Neck and back problems in adults with idiopathic scoliosis diagnosed in youth: An observational study of prevalence, change over a mean four year time period and comparison with a control group. *Scoliosis Spinal Disord,* 12, 1-7.
128. Dewan MC, Mummareddy N, Bonfield C (2018) The influence of pregnancy on women with adolescent idiopathic scoliosis. *Eur Spine J,* 27, 253-263.
129. Grabala P, Helenius I, Shah SA, et al. (2020) Impact of pregnancy on loss of deformity correction after pedicle screw instrumentation for adolescent idiopathic scoliosis. *World Neurosurg,* 139, 121-126.
130. Grabala P, Helenius I, Buchowski JM, Larson AN, Shah SA (2019) Back pain and outcomes of pregnancy after instrumented spinal fusion for adolescent idiopathic scoliosis. *World Neurosurg,* 124, 404-410.
131. Swany L, Larson AN, Shah SA, et al. (2020) Outcomes of pregnancy in operative vs. nonoperative adolescent idiopathic scoliosis patients at mean 30-year follow-up. *Spine Deform,* 8, 1169-1174.
132. Academy of Pediatric Physical Therapy (2019) Fact sheet: The ABCs of pediatric physical therapy. [pdf] Middleton WI, Academy of Pediatric Physical Therapy, Available at: <https://pediatricapta.org/includes/fact-sheets/pdfs/FactSheet_ABCs ofPediatricPT_2019.pdf?v=2> [Accessed April 24 2024].

Index

Figures and tables indicated by page numbers in italics.